MARKETING THE CONTINUUM OF CARE

Strategies for Developing Community Services

MARKETING THE CONTINUUM OF CARE

Strategies for Developing Community Services

VICKI MASON

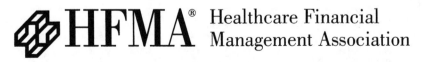

HFMA® Healthcare Financial Management Association

McGraw-Hill
New York   San Francisco   Washington, D.C.   Auckland   Bogotá
Caracas   Lisbon   London   Madrid   Mexico City   Milan
Montreal   New Delhi   San Juan   Singapore
Sydney   Tokyo   Toronto

McGraw-Hill

A Division of The McGraw-Hill Companies

1 2 3 4 5 6 7 8 9 0 BKM / BKM 9 0 9 8 7

ISBN 0-7863-1154-1

Printed and bound by Book-mart Press, Inc.

This publication is designed to provide accurate and authoritative information in regard to the
subject matter covered. It is sold with the understanding that neither the author nor
the publisher is engaged in rendering legal, accounting, or other professional service.
If legal advice or other expert assistance is required, the services of a competent professional
person should be sought.

> —*From a Declaration of Principles jointly adopted by a Committee of the American
> Bar Association and a Committee of Publishers.*

McGraw-Hill books are available at special quantity discounts to use as premiums and sales
promotions, or for use in corporate training programs. For more information, please write to
the Director of Sales, McGraw-Hill, 11 West 19th Street, New York, NY 10011. Or contact
your local bookstore.

Library of Congress Cataloging–in–Publication Data

Mason, Vicki
    Marketing the continuum of care : strategies for
developing community services / Vicki Mason.
        p.   cm.
    Includes index.
    ISBN 0-7863-1154-1
    1. Hospitals—Marketing.   2. Hospital and community.
3. Continuum of care.   I. Title.
RA965.5.M34   1997
362.1'1'0688—dc21   97-25979
                                                                    CIP

For those who gave me the chance to prove that I was equal to opportunity, Melinda Smolkin, Dan Flanagan, Jim Taylor, and Fred Fink. But most of all for the late Robert Gremore, who by his leadership and personal insights shared from his hospital bed, changed my life forever.

PREFACE

For far too long, many healthcare marketers have focused primarily on their own daily to-do list without solid understanding of the financial and clinical implications of the organization. Still others have lacked the in-depth knowledge to fully evaluate situations and creatively apply solutions. If the organization is to be successful in both developing new services and facilitating a seamless continuum delivery system, physicians and employees at all levels must understand the services available, have comprehensive knowledge about appropriate access, and fully support the system. Many organizations have invested resources in guest relations, recognition programs, and advertising, yet have seldom invested time in education about their own continuum of care services.

This book will serve as a reference for understanding target markets and potential promotional vehicles, as well as applying various marketing techniques creatively to components of the continuum.

ACKNOWLEDGMENTS

My thanks to the following contributors who shared their expertise for the benefit of all readers.

Jackie L. Anderson
Director of Marketing
Horizon Specialty Hospital
Horizon/CMS Health Care Corp.

William E. Brady
Regional Director of Operations
Prism Rehabilitation

Brad Buttry
Graphic Artist
Netlink Graphics

Godwin G. Dixon
Telesis Management

Sharla Findley
Director of Community Relations
Hillcrest Health Center

Connie Hawes
Manager, Customer Relations
Garland Community Hospital

Paula J. Lodes, MS, RN
Clinical Services
Health Care Development and Management
Netlink Health Systems, Inc.

Sandy Lutz
Former Southwestern Bureau Chief
Modern Healthcare

Cindy Long   Edward M. White
Community Relations Liaison   *Director, Managed Care*
North Texas Medical Center   *Private HealthCare Systems, Inc.*
Columbia Healthcare

Teri Webster, RN, MSN, MBA, NHA,
  CCM

But most of all to Janet Howe, Principal, Howe Communications of Dallas, Texas, whose contributions and editing gave thoughtful insight and new vision to this project.

C O N T E N T S

INTRODUCTION

Although the purpose of this book is to discuss marketing of the continuum components, a brief introduction to factors that have ultimately resulted in continuum and integrated delivery system (IDS) development is in order. These factors include:

- A decrease in acute care admissions, resulting in empty units. With managed care primarily driving decreased length of stay, admissions are often at higher level of acuity requiring intensive care and services (often resulting in DRG outliers and managed care contract losses).
- A need for more appropriate, cost-effective settings for delivery of quality care for the postacute patient—matching the level of service to the patient's needs and reducing "slippage" from the hospital or healthcare system when the service components are unavailable.
- Hospital, physician, management group and managed care competition for physicians, with new equipment, services, office buildings, medical directorships, and so on, as diverse providers and payors develop their continuums.
- Increased health education for the public driven by governmental studies, third parties, and consumer groups, resulting in consumer questions such as:

  "Why do I have to be in the hospital to get this service?"
  "What is it going to cost?"
  "If they don't have the service here, can I go to another hospital to get it?"

MANAGED CARE AS AN INFLUENCING FACTOR

The increasing influence of managed care and traditional indemnity insurers has spurred continuum development. For many healthcare organizations, the presence of a continuum of services facilitates competition for managed care contracts. In fact, many managed care organizations (MCOs), prefer to contract with hospitals or systems that offer a continuum rather than those that offer piecemeal services. (Refer to Chapter 18, Managed Care and Marketing Continuum). This preference is driven by:

- The overall managed care goal of changing practice patterns and patient choices, as well as the focus on provider management of care delivery at the most appropriate and efficient level of care
- The concept of disease state management now being employed by MCOs, and the focus of reducing costs by preventing illness and recidivism.

Managed care arrangements obligate providers to manage resources employed in the treatment of patients, much as Medicare diagnostic related groups (DRGs) have done. Responsibility is shifting increasingly. More insurers are actively directing their covered lives toward providers. The financial incentive for delivering quality care in the most cost-effective setting in and of itself is not bad. However, consumers need more education regarding their own care and providers need more education in optimizing their own delivery systems.

MEDICARE IMPACT

Many analysts might say, "As Medicare goes, so goes the direction of the business of healthcare." Consider that we are seeing a shift from acute care to postacute care for Medicare patients, and that Medicare spending on inpatient physical rehabilitation, home health, and skilled services has been increasing dramatically. Medicare is now allowing payment to physicians for management of home health care patients, and there is discussion of a need for a prospective payment system to be applied for outpatient services. Medicare and managed care trends are driving the current proliferation of cost-based programs as mechanisms for hospitals to provide more appropriate, cost-effective levels of care, to receive reimbursement for some of the hospital's overhead costs, and to reduce acute length of stay with effective use of alternative settings.

CONTINUUM OF CARE IMPLICATIONS

Those of us who began in healthcare as direct care providers are increasingly realizing that we have been very narrowly focused and task-oriented with relatively little knowledge of the big picture of healthcare delivery across the system. However, that orientation is changing. The most successful hospital departmental managers and marketers will be the ones who:

- Have an in-depth knowledge of reimbursement (Medicare and managed care)
- Be willing to learn more about the clinical delivery of care and to balance respect for established methods with the ability to question traditional assumptions
- Thoroughly evaluate and re-tool when necessary their approach to internal and external marketing expanding beyond discharge planning and product line management to managing the post-acute continuum process
- Educate medical staffs and hospital employees regarding the appropriate use of the continuum of care
- Ethically manage the continuum of care

Upcoming chapters will address areas within the continuum by diagnostic and related services, and a focus on linking components of the continuum for greater reader understanding. Creative methods within every diagnostic and service area for marketing to appropriate targets will be provided.

BUILDING AWARENESS
OF THE CONTINUUM

Part One of this book surveys services that may comprise a healthcare organization's continuum of care. More than just a listing, this section provides insight into disease incidence nationwide and the corresponding points of entry for continuum services. While the actual numbers are provided by national organizations, the prospective pathways are ours and should not be construed as reflective of any organization's strategies.

Part One focuses on the major categories of oncology, cardiac, diabetes, neurology and orthopedics (including arthritis). Major diagnostic group categories will vary from organization to organization, and every provider must identify and educate specifically on these groups. As marketers, we must have an understanding of different conditions and possible complications in order to envision the continuum of care possibilities.

Target markets and corresponding mechanisms for promotion to these groups also are included. It is our hope that they will offer the impetus for creative flow as readers see the potential to fine-tune their own marketing vehicles and use them across the continuum.

1

CHAPTER

An Overview of Continuum Components

This chapter will introduce some basic continuum service components, along with information about corresponding referral sources (see Figure 1–1). It is important that marketers understand the similarities and crossover among these components that may affect utilization, as well as their day-to-day continuum promotion.

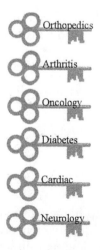

Orthopedics

Arthritis

Oncology

Diabetes

Cardiac

Neurology

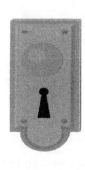

Skilled/Subacute Units
Acute Rehabilitation
Geropsychiatric Inpatient
Geropsychiatric Day Treatment
Cardiac Rehabilitation Outpatient
Physical Rehabilitation Outpatient
Home Health
Adult Day Care
Home Health
Long-Term Care
Assisted Living
Long-Term Care Hospital
Hospice

Figure 1–1

SKILLED/SUBACUTE (SHORT-TERM STAYS)

Referral Sources

Please note that although anyone can initiate a referral, only a physician can admit.

- Discharge planning professionals: social workers, utilization review/utilization management nurses, case managers
- Physicians
- Rehabilitation therapists (physical therapists, occupational therapists, speech therapists, and respiratory therapists)
- Nurses
- Managed care organizations

Patients and families will not generally be the drivers of this process but are more often educated by their discharge planning professional or physician. The gateway to skilled/subacute care is a three-day acute hospital stay within thirty days of admission to skilled care.

Promotional Avenues

- Usually one-to-one educational contacts
- Adjunct tools:
  Presentations and pocket cards for the medical staff on admitting and billing
  Stickers for charts or removable sticky notes from discharge planning professionals to encourage physicians to consider skilled nursing unit
  Office staff seminars on billing the SNU visit
  Continuum brochures in plastic holders on the backs of all hospital room doors
  In-service education for employees and presentations to physicians

Features and Benefits of Skilled/Subacute Care

Skilled/subacute care offers a bridge for discharges to home or to an alternative care setting and provides a cost-effective, quality environment. Medicare has established guidelines for admission, as follows: A three-day acute care hospital stay is required and admission to the skilled unit or facility must occur within thirty days of discharge from the acute hospital. If the patient meets criteria, services are covered by Medicare completely for the first twenty days. After twenty days the patient becomes responsible for daily co-payment.

There are basically five Medicare criteria for admission. The patient requires (1) skilled nursing and/or (2) skilled rehabilitation services daily. While most physicians and healthcare professionals understand skilled services and rehabilitation therapy, (3) observation and monitoring, (4) skilled teaching services, and (5) management and evaluation of the care plan may not be as familiar. This lack of familiarity may hamper appropriate admissions. This type of care is often an appropriate setting for many patients who are being referred to acute rehabilitation services but who need more time before they can tolerate the increased intensity. An acute rehabilitation patient (according to Medicare criteria, one who must be able to participate in three hours per day of therapy) and many older and more debilitated patients are simply not capable of this. The less intense setting allows patients to build up to the three hours of therapy. The skilled setting offers physicians the opportunity to continue to follow patients as they move out of the acute care setting to an alternative level of care.

There remains in many areas a lack of understanding of how often physicians may visit their patients in the skilled setting; this is an educational area to be emphasized. Also, because of many misconceptions regarding skilled care, providers are choosing to call their units "transitional care units" or "progressive care units," virtually anything *except* skilled units. Physician and employee misconceptions regarding the unit can significantly hamper the ramp up of the unit, and has done so in many facilities. Effective marketing and education about the unit conducted before it opens and soon after opening can alleviate this problem. An excellent resource for information on this continuum service is the American Subacute Care Association at (305) 864-0396.

ACUTE REHABILITATION
Referral Sources

Please note that although anyone can refer only a physician can admit.

- Discharge planning professionals: social workers, UR nurses, case managers

- Nurses, therapists and other hospital-based employees
- Physicians
- Managed care organizations
- Physician office staffs
- Home health direct care providers and home care coordinators
- Nursing homes
- Families and patients
- General public (groups and social organizations, clergy, support groups, volunteers, and individuals)

Promotional Avenues

- To physicians, managed care organizations, and all hospital-based professionals

  One-to-one educational contacts (especially effective is the physician medical director to physicians and insurers)

  Continuing education, grand rounds, case study presentations

- To Physicians

  Small pocket cards to explain admitting criteria and billing information

- To Families and Patients

  Continuum brochures in plastic holders on the backs of patient room doors

  Direct mail to those individuals who have been discharged with diagnoses that often benefit from rehab services but who do not appear in rehab admissions, information regarding support groups, and so on

  Public campaign direct mail or health fairs: "Have you or someone you love lost the ability to . . ."

- To Home Health Representatives

  In-service education to teach caregivers to focus on an individual's loss of function and to identify patients who may benefit from rehab and return to home care after discharge

- To Nursing Homes
  One-to-one contacts with therapists, nurses, and social workers. This is more successful when the nursing home does not offer interdisciplinary treatment teams and the acute rehabilitation program is not considered to be competition. Often patients who appear to have little potential for improvement (and therefore do not qualify for acute rehabilitation services) are placed in a nursing home and later begin to progress. The patient can then qualify for acute rehabilitation services.
- To the general public
  Some hospitals have used TV, radio, and print effectively to demonstrate the continuum of care for stroke.

Features and Benefits of Acute Rehabilitation

The gateway to acute rehabilitation is usually an acute care stay via acute hospital or skilled unit, although there are cases of admitting patients from home when they meet criteria, including the following. In addition to the qualifying diagnoses, the patient must require twenty-four-hour physician and RN availability, with therapy three hours a day, five days a week with a multidisciplinary team approach. The patient must be medically stable and possess mental alertness to participate in the rehab program. There must be significant improvement expected in a reasonable period of time. Patients must be unable to function independently with impairments within one of the following: self-care, cognitive or perceptual function, mobility, continence, communication, and pain management. Commercial insurors and managed care organizations often have their own criteria, with a preadmission verification of benefits and authorization for the admission necessary. The American Rehabilitation Association in Reston, Virginia, at (800) 368-3513 is an excellent resource for this type of program, as well as for outpatient rehabilitation programs.

The Health Care Financing Administration (HCFA) has set forth guidelines on Medicare coverage for acute rehabilitation services that specify diagnoses and corresponding DRGs. The peer review organization (PRO) in your particular state is the best resource; there can be differences in how PROs interpret the list.

INPATIENT GEROPSYCHIATRIC PROGRAMS

Referral Sources

Please note that in most programs only a psychiatrist evaluates the patient for the appropriateness of an inpatient admission. Anyone can make a referral but the patient must be screened and approved by a physician.

- Discharge planning professionals: social workers, UR nurses, case managers
- Physicians (The primary referral sources for such programs are often primary care physicians and internists)
- Physician office staff
- Families
- Employers (via employee assistance plans [EAPs])
- Nursing homes, adult day care, assisted living, and retirement communities
- Agencies and organizations that act as community resources and maintain lists of programs
- Clergy
- Attorneys and trust officers

Promotional Avenues

One-to-one education is the best way to address the complexities of the admission criteria. Printed materials must be concise and must direct the individual considering a referral to place a call for more information. It is also helpful if the medical director of the program talks with other physicians who could refer.

Features and Benefits of Inpatient Geropsychiatric Programs

These types of programs provide hospital-based care to older persons in need of intensive psychiatric treatment, and although somewhat controversial, some indicate that this may be an appropriate setting for ECT. There must be documented criteria present for admission such as severe uncontrolled behavior with risk of harm to others or oneself, anxiety disorders, uncontrollable behavior, or severe depression. As with acute rehabilitation programs, the patient must be able to participate;

extreme confusion, delirium, or terminal status are contraindicated. The programs usually feature an interdisciplinary approach to the total care of the patient. Professionals include: a psychiatrist, a physician to follow the medical needs of the patient, social worker, nurses, occupational therapists, psychologists and activity/recreational specialists. The complexity of medical needs and medication monitoring in some elderly persons may be more suited for twenty-four-hour-a-day inpatient care rather than outpatient programs. Family counseling and involvement are often an important component to such programs. The goal of inpatient geropsychiatric programs is to provide patients with their highest possible level of emotional, social, and physical independence. The individual's mental state may actually impair their abilities for self-care, so the approach is behavioral and therapeutic. Many family members will select a hospital-based unit and emphasize the acute care setting in lieu of freestanding facilities. As stated with skilled units, the trend is toward using euphemisms for naming these units, so that patients will be on the "Senior Care" or "Geriatric Behavioral Unit," with no psychiatric reference. Some hospitals have experienced long ramp up periods of six months to one year for these types of units, attributed to the combination of perceptions about mental health and the complexities of admissions criteria.

DAY TREATMENT GEROPSYCHIATRIC PROGRAMS
Referral Sources

Please note that although anyone may initiate a referral, the decision of patient appropriateness for admission is made by a physician, usually a psychiatrist.

- Inpatient geropsychiatric programs
- Physicians (most often primary care and psychiatrists)
- Nursing homes
- Outpatient rehabilitation units
- Family
- Discharge planning professionals
- Agencies and organizations
- Clergy
- Physician office staff

Promotional Avenues

- Usually one-to-one educational contacts are the most effective with this complex product.

Features and Benefits of Geropsychiatric Partial Day Treatment Programs

The individual may receive care during the day and return home (home or a nursing home) in the evening. It is an alternative to inpatient hospitalization and is appropriate for many persons who do not require inpatient care. As in inpatient programs, services offered include mental health treatment, therapeutic intervention, medical services, education, and family services. Many of these programs provide transportation for participants. A resource for this programmatic area is the American Association for Partial Hospitalization in Alexandria, Virginia, at (703) 836-2274.

OUTPATIENT CARDIAC REHABILITATION PROGRAMS

Referral Sources

Please note that although anyone may initiate a referral, only a physician can admit.

- Physicians (cardiologists, internists)
- Discharge planning professionals: Social workers, UR nurses, case managers
- Unit nursing staff (coronary care unit [CCU], step down, telemetry)
- Managed care organizations that focus on wellness and preventing recidivism
- Physician office staffs
- Patients and families
- General public

Promotional Avenues

- One-to-one educational contacts to health care professionals, physicians and managed care organizations

- Seminars and educational presentations to hospital-based professionals
- Payroll stuffers
- Office staff education
- Physician office brochures for patient education
- Direct mail to patients discharged from acute care within allowable DRGs
- Cardiology continuum brochures in plastic holders on the back of patient room doors in appropriate units, CCU waiting areas, and so on.

Features and Benefits of Cardiac Rehabilitation Programs

These programs are excellent for many patients (angioplasty, angina, heart attack, or bypass surgery) who wish to take more responsibility for their condition and make lifestyle changes. Medicare has very clear guidelines for admissions including: myocardial infarct (MI) within the preceding twelve months, coronary artery bypass graft (CABG) or angina. A patient is limited to thirty-six sessions in a lifetime, unless there is a subsequent MI or CABG. The patient must be clinically stable to participate. While some insurance programs have similar guidelines, every insurer is different. Programs must verify insurance coverage. Documentation and tests required for admission vary somewhat by individual program. Cardiac rehabilitation programs usually feature nurses, dietitians, and exercise physiology professionals, with both exercise and education components. The education involves risk factors, proper diet, and how to monitor the response to exercise and activity. Exercise is both supervised and monitored to improve capacity and endurance gradually.

OUTPATIENT PHYSICAL REHABILITATION PROGRAMS

Referral Sources

Please note that although anyone may refer a patient, treatment is by physician's order.

- Inpatient physical rehabilitation programs
- Inpatient geropsychiatric programs
- Physicians

- Managed care organizations
- Private medical case managers
- Employers
- Schools (pediatric patients)
- Physician office staffs
- Nursing homes
- Home health agencies
- Patients and family
- General public

Promotional Avenues

- One-to-one direct educational contacts
- Radio, outdoor, and print media

The patient's choice of a provider often centers on location and convenience, so marketing directly to the patient becomes more important and cost effective.

Features and Benefits of Outpatient Physical Rehabilitation Programs

Outpatient rehab services may be an alternative or follow-up to inpatient rehabilitation services and are appropriate for many persons who do not require twenty-four-hour care. The services can be offered through Comprehensive Outpatient Rehabilitation Facilities (CORFs), a Medicare cost-based program. These are reimbursed as Medicare Part B services. A CORF may offer a variety of services including physician, nursing, social work, therapy (physical, occupational, and respiratory), home evaluation, psychiatric, drugs, equipment, and supplies, and prosthetics. Services for younger patients may be specialized through physical therapy, hand therapy, or industrial or sports medicine clinics. Flexible treatment hours and days of service including weekends and transportation are selling points. Regardless of the setting, the focus is to assist the individual in achieving the highest possible level of functioning and independence. The American Rehabilitation Association in Reston, Virginia, at (800) 368-3513 is a resource.

HOME HEALTH CARE SERVICES

Referral Sources

Please note that although anyone may refer a patient, service may only begin by physician order.

- Discharge planners
- Physicians
- Managed care organizations
- General public

Promotional Avenues

- One-to-one educational contacts
- Educational forums
- Health fairs
- Presentations and mailings to physicians regarding billing for oversight of home care plan

Features and Benefits of Home Health Care

Home care is often the appropriate delivery setting for infirm or elderly individuals who cannot avail themselves of outpatient care or for those who wish to remain within their own homes. A hospital or healthcare organization can reach out to patients through its home care program. A wide variety of services are available through the home care service and may include AIDS care, postobstetrical (maternal-child), pediatric, cardiac, IV infusion, pulmonary, cancer, diabetes, rehabilitation, palliative care, and wound care, among many others. Types of patients visited varies by each home care provider organization, according to patient diagnoses and demographics, and other continuum components available within the market. According to the National Association for Home Care (NAHC) publication *Basic Statistics about Home Care 1996*, 26.3 percent of home health patients have cardiac diagnoses, 8.4 percent have musculoskeletal diagnoses, and 6.5 percent have neoplasms and the nervous system disorders. It says that the five DRGs most likely to result in home care utilization are DRG 14 stroke; 88 COPD, 127 heart failure, 209 major joint procedures, and 210 hip/femur procedures. Home health services are also Medicare cost-based programs, although not all home health care agencies are Medicare certified. Many managed care organizations cover home health care when they do not offer benefits for care in other settings. A resource is the National Association for Home Care in Washington, D.C., at (202) 547-7424.

ADULT DAY CARE PROGRAMS

Referral Sources

Please note that although anyone may refer a patient, service may only begin by physician order.

- Discharge planners
- Physicians
- Senior assistance organizations
- Clergy
- General public

Promotional Avenues

- One-to-one educational contacts
- Health fairs
- Presentations
- Mailings to senior advocacy organizations
- Advertisement in senior publications and other print media
- Human interest stories in print media

Features and Benefits of Adult Day Care

Individuals who require less than twenty-four-hour care can often benefit from adult day care programs. These programs vary widely in their setting from hospital based programs, nursing or assisted living facility–based or freestanding programs. They also vary in their focus. One may choose from programs developed for persons with Alzheimer's disease, dementia, and other memory problems, or programs for those with no cognitive difficulties. These programs differ from simply taking one's loved one to a senior center in that there are often security systems, more medical personnel on-site (to supervise medication administration, monitor medical needs, conduct therapy sessions, etc.), and regularly scheduled visits from ancillary providers such as dentists or podiatrists. Some programs provide transportation within boundaries for a fee; others provide no transportation at all. Hours vary from site to site, with some facilities open up to twelve hours per day. Most have core hours from 9 or 10 a.m. until 3 or 4 p.m. Adult day care programs often offer a light breakfast snack, lunch, and afternoon snack, plus activities throughout the day. Many programs even offer "shower hours," opportunities to help those individuals who may need assistance in bathing, grooming, and hygiene. Some programs feature caregiver sessions with guest speakers to build a better understanding for different conditions. Adult day care programs seem to be proliferating in many areas of the country and filling a gap in the healthcare system. The services are private pay, covered by some state Medicaid programs, and some long term care policies. Medicare does not cover this service. The National Adult Day Service Association at (202) 479-6682 is a resource for this continuum component.

LONG-TERM CARE SPECIALTY HOSPITALS

Referral Sources

Please note that although anyone can refer, only a physician can admit.

- Discharge planning professionals: social workers, UR nurses, case managers
- Nurses, therapists, and other hospital-based employees
- Physicians
- Managed care organizations
- Physician office staffs
- Home health direct care providers and home care coordinators
- Nursing homes
- Families and patients
- General public (groups and social organizations, clergy, support groups, volunteers, and individuals)

Promotional Avenues

- To physicians and their office staffs
  One-to-one education contacts
  Luncheons
  Case studies
- To healthcare professionals
  One-to-one education contacts
  Case study collaterals and presentations
- To the general public
  Human interest stories
  Radio and television talk shows with physicians
  Print media advertisements
  Public education presentations

Features and Benefits of Long-Term Care Specialty Hospitals

These facilities are licensed as hospitals, with the specialty hospital designation for a length of stay over twenty-five days (long-term acute). Referral targets are virtually the same as those for acute rehabilitation: the majority of patients come from the acute hospital setting through discharge planners and physicians. Patients are admitted from home as well, although in smaller proportions. These patients are post–intensive care unit patients who are stable and can be transferred. The patients are the medically complex, and/or rehabilitation candidates. Specialty hospitals may include services such as telemetry, dialysis, and ventilators that are not routinely found in other postacute settings. A resource in this area of the continuum is the Long Term Acute Care Hospital Association of America at (202) 296-4446.

ASSISTED LIVING

Referral Sources

- Social workers/discharge planning professionals
- Physicians and their office staffs.
- General public

- Volunteers
- Visiting entertainers
- Church groups
- Social organization
- Support groups
  Respite Care
- Travel Agents
- Social service organizations
- Churches

Promotional Avenues

- One-to-one contacts
- Advertising in print and broadcast media
- Videos
- Mailings to senior advocacy organizations
- Public presentations

Features and Benefits of Assisted Living

The number of assisted living facilities is rapidly growing to meet the needs of the aging population. These programs are usually self- or private-pay programs, but are covered by Medicaid in a few states. Correspondingly, types of facilities range from those with the basic comforts to the very luxurious. The American Health Care Association's *Facts: Assisted Living Quick Reference* offers this definition: "Assisted living is part of a comprehensive long term care continuum that provides the necessary level of services to dependent elderly or disabled population in the appropriate environment. Assisted living services include: 24 hour protective oversight, food, shelter, and the provision and/or coordination of a range of services that promote the quality of life of the individual."[1] The association also says that staffing may include personal care attendants, administrators, activities coordinators, maintenance personnel, food service managers, and nurses. These programs can vary from small suites (much like efficiency apartments) in mid- or high-rise buildings to small cottages. The individual retains a "private" residence and facility representatives, caregivers, housekeepers, and so on enter the residence to assist the individual. Programs differ in the level of assistance available. Some services may be added to the basic package. The individual may have limited kitchen facilities or may take all of their meals in the community dining room. A variety of activities are provided and may include transportation services. Providers are partnering with vendors in rehabilitation, hospice services, home health, pharmacy, and medical supplies, as well as with such providers as beauticians and podiatrists, to facilitate a more comprehensive offering to their residents. Some assisted living providers offer adult day care programs on site. Not only does this generate revenue, but also serves to market the facility for future residents. The final admission decision is generally driven by family members and the individual. The Assisted Living Federation of America in Fairfax, Virginia, at (703) 691-8100 is a resource for this continuum product.

LONG-TERM CARE NURSING FACILITIES

Referral Sources

- Discharge planning professionals: social workers, UR nurses, case managers
- Nurses, therapists, and other hospital-based employees
- Physicians and physician office staffs
- Home health
- Acute rehabilitation programs
- Inpatient geropsychiatric programs
- Specialty hospitals
- Families and patients
- General public (groups and social organizations, clergy, support groups, volunteers, and individuals)

Promotional Avenues

- One-to-one direct contacts
- Health fairs

- Human interest stories to senior publications
- Print advertising

Features and Benefits of Long-Term Care Nursing Facilities

Long-term care has been making a transition in many areas of the country from maintenance to both restorative and maintenance. (Refer to our information on skilled/subacute units). Facilities are adding skilled units, specialty care units, and other complimentary programs such as home health, adult day care, hospice, assisted living, and outpatient rehabilitation services to develop their own continuums of care and generate revenue. Many organizations now have campuses centered on long-term facilities. Long-term care or that which is maintenance in nature and does not meet skilled care criteria is funded by Medicaid after an individual qualifies financially. The American Health Care Association's *Facts: Today's Nursing Homes and the People They Serve* uses HCFA figures in separating nursing home residents by primary payor source: 68.7 percent are Medicaid and 23.5 percent are private pay/other. Medicaid coverage is usually after a "spend down" with only a specified asset amount remaining. If an individual has assets and does not qualify for Medicaid, the care is not funded by Medicaid and the individual is referred to as "private pay." There is of course, insurance available that covers costs associated with long-term care. A resource is the American Healthcare Association in Washington, D.C., at (202) 842-4444.

HOSPICE

Referral Sources

Please note that although anyone may initiate a referral, service may begin only by physician order.

- Discharge planners
- Physicians
- Nursing homes
- Home health agencies
- Clergy

- Managed care organizations
- General public

Promotional Avenues

- One-to-one educational contacts on referral sources
- Health fairs
- Presentations and mailings to health care professionals

Features and Benefits of Hospice Programs

Hospices provide palliative care to the terminally ill. The patient receiving such services has a life expectancy of less than six months. According to the Hospice Association of America in *Hospice Facts and Statistics 1995*, services include nursing, medical social worker, physician, counselor (dietary, pastoral, and other), home care aide and homemaker, short-term inpatient care (including both respite care and procedures necessary for pain control and acute and chronic system management), medical appliances and supplies including drugs and biologicals, physical and occupational therapies, and speech language pathology services. Bereavement service for a family is provided for up to thirteen months following the patient's death. The association reports that 71.5 percent of hospice patients are 65 years of age and over. The report cites a recent survey by the National Center for Health Statistics in stating that 71 percent of patients have diagnoses of neoplasms and 9 percent have circulatory system diagnoses. Hospice benefits are covered by Medicare, but not every hospice is Medicare certified. There are three benefit periods for the Medicare hospice benefit after the initial ninety-day period. They include a subsequent ninety-day period, a subsequent thirty-day period, and a fourth and final indefinite duration period. A resource in this area of the continuum is the Hospice Association of America in Washington, D.C., at (202) 546-4759.

REFERENCE

1. American Health Care Association. Facts: Assisted living quick reference.

2

CHAPTER

Oncology Services

In *Cancer Facts and Figures 1997* the American Cancer Society (ACS) estimates that there will be 1,382,400 new cancer cases within the year.[1] Figure 2–1 shows the number of ACS listed cases. We have taken these statistics and interpreted them into a continuum-friendly format.

As you might surmise, costs associated with care of these patients is staggering. According to the ACS, "The National Cancer Institute estimates overall costs for cancer at $104 billion; $35 billion for direct medical costs" and further states that "over half of the direct medical costs are due to the treatment of breast cancer, lung cancer and prostate cancer."[1]

As patients progress through acute care continuums, they pass through diagnostic and cancer treatment services, as well as inpatient care as needed.

For some patients, the diagnosis of cancer may be a chance situation, after a routine physician visit for a pap smear or during a screening clinic sponsored by a hospital as a public service. For others, it may follow a period of ill health or indications that a serious problem exists. A patient may have already visited a physician a number of times and entered our continuum in the diagnostics services component of the system. Hospitals have long recognized the special needs of cancer diagnosis and treatment and the impact they can have on the facility's financial performance. Think of the hospitals in your areas that long ago proactively developed their cancer treatment centers and specialty oncology units. These oncology programs have tied together the service components of diagnostics, surgery, and therapy (both in radiation and

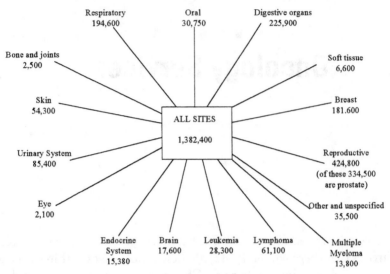

Figure 2–1 Estimated New Cancer Cases 1997[1]

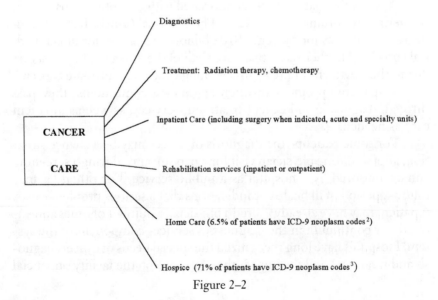

Figure 2–2

chemotherapy). Nurses received special education and the designation "oncology nurse" or "clinical nurse specialist in oncology." State-of-the-art linear accelerators were installed and outpatient chemotherapy areas developed within hospitals' ambulatory treatment centers. It seemed that our continuum was complete. But how times have changed.

Next, freestanding rehabilitation centers and acute hospital rehab units began to develop "oncology rehabilitation programs," and we began to read published articles on how these services could affect the quality of life of cancer survivors. Our paradigm of removing and treating the cancer as the completion of treatment was suddenly and irreversibly altered. Oncologists and surgeons were being asked to consider that the treatment was not finished but in some aspects just begun. This was a slow education process for many reasons. It involved not only expanding our way of thinking about cancer and the needs of cancer patients but also introducing services with cancer patients that had been traditionally associated with other types of patients (rehabilitation associated with stroke and trauma, for example). Now these patients may move through our continuum. They may need skilled services to do so, to learn to care for their new colostomy or for the management of pain medications as part of their care plan. What about rehabilitation or home health services? Can they swallow after their radiation therapy or chemotherapy? What is their nutritional status as a result of the chemotherapy or radiation? Could they benefit from sessions with a dietitian in our outpatient facility? What about sessions with a psychologist or social worker to cope with the life changes brought about by cancer? Do they need the services of a speech therapist after a laryngectomy?

After their cancer treatment, many patients still experience the effects of cancer and its treatment. Beside the emotional toll, they are likely to experience debilitation from surgery, therapy, or both. Our challenge is to determine the scope of their needs and provide assistance. Depending on the primary or metastatic site and treatment involved, patients may have problems with mobility, incontinence, decreased ability to perform the activities of daily living such as bathing, grooming, or dressing or have difficulty swallowing. They may be appropriate for our acute rehab units because of loss of a limb or metastatic cancer pressing on their spinal cord, resulting in paralysis.

Their physical condition after the surgery or treatment may well dictate in which setting they are best served. Their finances and insurance coverage may make this decision for them.

But with continuum services in place, treatment is provided in the most appropriate setting for these patients, who in many cases are simply focused on going home and returning to some degree of normality within their lives.

Our challenge is to assist these persons in their recovery by providing knowledge of and access to all necessary continuum components, while simultaneously educating those referral sources who neither understand nor believe that further services can be beneficial. The education of healthcare professionals can be the most challenging, as many of them believe that nothing more is beneficial once the cancer is addressed. Many persons need more than time to recover to their fullest potential, and we have the services to offer. As marketers, can we teach people to think outside of the box the healthcare delivery system has created?

Consider that the incidence of cancer rises with age—and the baby boomers are aging. The size of this demographic group as it approaches retirement age is astounding. Concurrently, managed care is continuing to proliferate. What does this mean to hospitals and other healthcare organizations? First, if we extrapolate, the percentage of cancer as a diagnosis within the profile of each of our hospitals and organizations could begin to grow. Early detection will become more and more important. It will become important first to the patients as more people enter the risk groups for development of cancer. The baby boomer generation is more attuned to the risk of cancer than previous generations. This has occurred through the enhanced education efforts of groups like the American Cancer Society. This means that as marketers, we will consider more screening events and public education. Prevention and early detection will become more important to hospitals and payors because it is more cost-effective, and more likely to cure the cancer, when treatment is begun early. The highest costs, to providers and payors, will be surgery and treatment of the cancer. If we can affect these types of costs, we can become more efficient in managing the bottom line. Currently, the cost of cancer is estimated to be $104 billion and this cost will grow in proportion to the aging of the population. Thus, it will become imperative to move these patients efficiently and effectively through our continuum of care not only to prevent recidivism but to preserve our own financial health.

I. Target Groups
  A. Physicians
  B. Hospital-based employees
  C. General public
II. Mechanisms
  A. Physicians
    1. Office staff education events
    2. One-to-one educational contacts
    3. Presentations to/with the medical staff on "continuum case studies"
    4. Medical Director of cancer treatment center networking with other medical staff members
    5. Articles in medical staff newsletter
  B. Hospital-based employees
    1. Case study brown bag or luncheon events
    2. Articles in hospital or facility newsletter
    3. Payroll stuffers
    4. Tours
    5. Multimedia presentations
    6. Educational vehicles provided by vendors (equipment and drug)
  C. General public
    1. Radio and television talk shows with physician experts
    2. Articles placed in newspapers or senior publications
    3. Human interest stories in the print and broadcast media
    4. Screening events
      a. Mammography
      b. Colon-rectal screenings
      c. Prostate screenings
    5. Educational seminars
    6. Health fairs
    7. Sponsorships and participation in educational opportunities (such as fun runs and other sporting events)

SUMMARY

For this patient population, the diagnosis of cancer is often just the entry into the continuum of care. The residual effects of cancer and cancer treatment often necessitate postacute services that can improve quality of life. In Chapter 20, "The Marketer's Toolbox," we have included examples of promotional strategies including the continuum of care case study, educational seminars, and brown bag luncheon series, as well as others that may be creatively tailored to your needs.

REFERENCES

1. American Cancer Society 1997. Cancer facts and figures, p. 1, 3, 4.
2. National Association for Home Care, September 1996. Basic statistics about home care.
3. The Hospice Association of America 1995. Hospice facts and statistics 1995.

3 CHAPTER

Orthopedic and Arthritis Services

For many healthcare providers, an orthopedic continuum of care will be the most likely first step in continuum development, because combining existing services into a continuum will enhance the individual components of the product line. This will be a shift from the "heads in beds" mentality that some hospitals demonstrated in the past. The discharge planning effort will become one of facilitating flow into the most appropriate care setting.

Consider these statistics on fractures from the American Academy of Orthopedic Surgeons' Department of Research and Scientific Affairs:[1]

- Approximately 6.5 million fractures occur each year in the United States.
- More than 900,000 hospitalizations result each year from fractures.
- In 1993, fractures most frequently resulting in hospitalization were those of the hip (307,000), ankle (111,000), and tibia and fibula (79,000).
- More than half (52 percent) of fractures resulting in hospitalization occur in persons age 65 and over, including

90 percent of hip fractures, 65 percent of pelvic fractures, and 49 percent of vertebral fractures.

- In 1993, more than 4.2 million fractures were seen by physicians in office-based practices.

Orthopedics generally has a long life cycle from a marketing standpoint, because orthopedic patients are likely to need services on an intermittent and ongoing basis. This is largely due to the types of diagnoses and conditions, such as arthritis and chronic pain. But even an elderly person who has sustained a hip fracture and undergone surgery is likely to continue to experience difficulties or have concurrent conditions that may indicate a need for skilled nursing, physical rehabilitation (inpatient or outpatient), or home healthcare. Many of these persons are also predisposed to future joint problems that may necessitate additional surgeries.

According to the American Academy of Orthopedic Surgeons in *Live It Safe:*[2]

- More than 280,000 people suffer hip fractures each year.
- The total cost in medical bills and lost income resulting from hip fractures is more than $9.8 billion a year or an average of $35,000 per hip fracture.
- Because of the aging U.S. population, the number of hip fractures is expected to reach about 350,000 a year by the year 2000.
- Most hip fracture patients who previously lived independently will require home care or assistance from their families.
- Forty percent of hip fracture patients 65 and older are discharged from hospitals to long-term care facilities.
- All hip fracture patients require walking aids for several months after injury, and nearly half will permanently require canes or walkers.

These figures indicate the need for postacute care, to move successfully to home or to an alternative level of care. These patients may travel through our continuum receiving services from multiple components as illustrated in Figure 3–1.

Some of these hip fractures may occur as a result of arthritis. Because arthritis is in most cases a chronic condition, these individuals are likely to move in and out of the continuum, through remissions

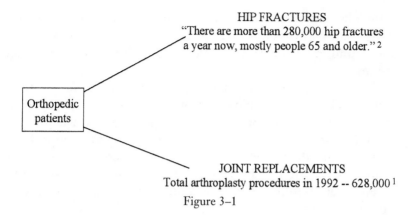

HIP FRACTURES
"There are more than 280,000 hip fractures
a year now, mostly people 65 and older." 2

Orthopedic
patients

JOINT REPLACEMENTS
Total arthroplasty procedures in 1992 -- 628,000 1

Figure 3-1

and flare-ups. The Arthritis Foundation reports in the booklet *Arthritis Information: Basic Facts: Answers to Your Questions,* "The key is in getting proper medical help early in the course of the disease and in faithfully staying with the treatment program even during remissions".3 In the case of the arthritis patient's safety, joint protection and energy conservation techniques may dramatically reduce recidivism and are a wise investment of time. But that time no longer need be spent in a bed. They may move through different continuum settings while the joint is repaired (see Figure 3-2).

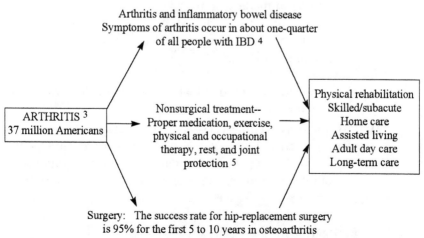

Arthritis and inflammatory bowel disease
Symptoms of arthritis occur in about one-quarter
of all people with IBD 4

ARTHRITIS 3
37 million Americans

Nonsurgical treatment--
Proper medication, exercise,
physical and occupational
therapy, rest, and joint
protection 5

Physical rehabilitation
Skilled/subacute
Home care
Assisted living
Adult day care
Long-term care

Surgery: The success rate for hip-replacement surgery
is 95% for the first 5 to 10 years in osteoarthritis

Figure 3-2

Providing access to treatment and education throughout the levels of the continuum allows the individual to take control of their own healthcare and to live more successfully within the limitations of their condition.

While our marketing strategies can attract more new patients and build market share, keeping them within the continuum is a complicated process. It is important to know the target groups for marketing and to develop techniques to educate effectively, and to facilitate continuum flow. Seminars, screening events, preadmission programs, and continuum brochures are excellent tools available for marketers in promoting orthopedic continuum services. We have included samples in Chapter 20, "The Marketer's Toolbox."

Few hospital marketers believe that an opening event, no matter how well done, ensures referrals. It is the wiser one who knows that the key is education. A "field of dreams" concept will not necessarily result in referrals; just because you build it doesn't mean they will come. Unfortunately, while some will spend large sums on advertising campaigns, our internal referral sources and salespeople are often overlooked in the hospital sales campaign. And so the most immediate group available to promote our services at little incremental costs remain unable to promote our own continuum effectively.

Target Groups

  I. Physicians
    A. Articles in medical staff newsletter
    B. Presentations to medical staff or section groups
    C. One-to-one educational contacts
    D. Grand rounds
    E. Case studies
    F. Development of individual protocols for postacute care of their patients

  II. Hospital-based employees—Nurses, therapists, discharge planning professionals, x-ray and laboratory technologists, and so on. These people have daily contact with patients and physicians and are influencers in the sales process at the very least.
    A. Articles in hospital newsletter
    B. Payroll stuffers
    C. In-house education seminars
    D. Departmental presentations

    E. Tours
    F. Multimedia displays
    G. Spotlight on different healthcare recognition and event
        days using the American Hospital Association's calendar
III. General public
    A. Free public education seminars
    B. Radio and print ads
    C. American Academy of Orthopedic Surgeons in
        Rosemont, Ill. ("Play It Safe," "Live It Safe," and
        "Drive It Safe")
    D. Arthritis Foundation in the local area
    E. Joint replacement seminars
    F. Arthritis screenings with physicians
    G. Media features: Human interest stories for radio,
        television, and print

SUMMARY

If you are not a clinician, go to the library or to national organizations to increase your knowledge of different areas that include the major proportion of diagnoses at your hospital or organization. Spend time speaking with direct caregivers within your own organization who can impart to you a broader understanding of patients' needs. Effective promotion is easier when you have a clear understanding of the product and its benefits. We have included specific strategies—such as joint replacement seminars, elective orthopedic preadmission programs, an orthopedic continuum of care brochure outline, arthritis and hand screenings, and arthritis education outlines—within Chapter 20, "The Marketer's Toolbox."

REFERENCES

1. The American Academy of Orthopaedic Surgeons 1996. Summary data on fractures.
2. American Academy of Orthopaedic Surgeons 1992. Live it safe.
3. Arthritis Foundation 1992. Arthritis information: Basic facts, p. 4.
4. Arthritis Foundation 1992. Arthritis information: Arthritis inflammatory bowel disease, pp. 1-9.
5. Arthritis Foundation 1992. Arthritis information: Surgery: Information to consider, p. 1, 11.

4
CHAPTER

Diabetes Services

The sheer percentage of the population with diabetes (both diagnosed and undiagnosed) is staggering. *In Diabetes Facts and Figures,* the American Diabetes Association states that 5 percent of the U.S. population, or more than 13 million people, have diabetes. Of those individuals, only about 7 million have been diagnosed. Because diabetes is a process disorder, these individuals face an extraordinary challenge in taking responsibility for managing their condition.[1]

Diabetes treatment services are another example of long product life cycle. This patient population is seriously at risk for a multitude of complications and could benefit from an ongoing relationship with healthcare providers (both physicians and facilities). Perhaps more than other patients, they can be served well by educational approaches. Again, please note that the potential continuum services illustration in Figure 4–1 is strictly our representation of the marketer's conceptual approach to continuum understanding and promotion and is not endorsed by any organization.

The longer a person has had diabetes, the higher the risk for developing diabetic neuropathy.[2] Neuropathy is damage to the nerves and can affect many different parts of the body. It causes a loss in sensation. This means that an individual can have a developing problem

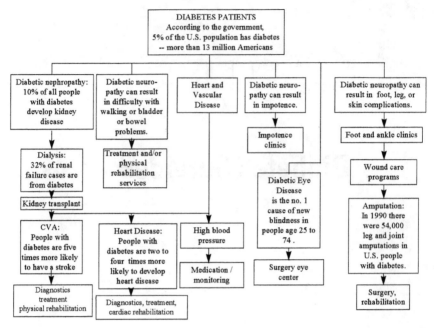

Figure 4–1

and be unaware of it. Although a neuropathy may affect different areas, many healthcare professionals immediately associate foot problems with diabetics. Many organizations have created foot and ankle clinics, along with wound care centers, as components of diabetes treatment centers. Because of the nerve and vascular complications that many diabetics may experience, any skin problem can result in a crisis. The nerve and vascular damage prevent skin from healing. The condition can progress and result in amputation. Wound care clinics treat nonhealing areas and attempt to prevent further skin breakdown.

Nerve or blood vessel damage can also cause impotence in diabetic men.[3] Treatment of the diabetes, surgery, or implants may address the condition.[4] Impotence clinics are helpful to these types of patients.

Figure 4–1 notes that people with diabetes are two to four times more likely to develop heart disease. They are also likely to do so at an earlier age.[5] An individual may enter a different component of the continuum of care with a cardiac episode or a stroke from high blood pressure.

Another condition that may affect persons with diabetes is kidney disease or nephropathy.[6] We often associate kidney disease with older diabetics. As noted in Figure 4–1, 10 percent of all people with diabetes develop kidney disease. Some of these patients will require dialysis. Hospitals with a significant population of diabetes diagnoses have implemented dialysis services to expand their continuum services. Transplants may be indicated for some of these patients.

Diabetic retinopathy affects the retina of the eye. There are two types of retinopathy. Background retinopathy occurs in about half of all people with diabetes after they have had the disease for 10 to 15 years. If left untreated it can cause a more serious type of retinopathy, proliferative retinopathy and lead to blindness. Diabetics also develop cataracts earlier than other people and they are most likely to develop glaucoma.[7] Eye clinics may be part of this continuum product.

This information illustrates how the direct and indirect costs for diabetes can mount—to nearly $92 billion annually and to nearly 6 percent of total U.S. healthcare costs.[1]

I. Target groups
   A. Physicians
   B. Hospital-based employees
   C. General public
II. Mechanisms
   A. Physicians
      1. One-to-one educational contacts with case studies
      2. Office staff education events
      3. "Continuum case studies"
   B. Hospital-based employees
      1. "Continuum case studies" brown bag or luncheon events
      2. Articles in hospital newsletter
      3. Payroll stuffers
   C. General public
      1. Radio and television talk shows, news features
      2. Human interest stories with sidebars on the disease placed in newspapers or senior publications
      3. Screening events (blood sugars)
      4. Associated clinics (never compete with your medical staff)

        a. Eye clinics
        b. Incontinence clinics
        c. Impotence clinics
        d. Wound care clinics
        e. Nutrition clinics
        f. Exercise clinics
        g. Foot and ankle clinics
   5. Diet-related courses, everything from supermarket
      shopping education and tours to courses on losing or
      maintaining weight sensibly
III. The Message
   A. To Physicians
      1. The diabetes program augments your care; it does
         not replace it.
      2. Professionals in the diabetes program offer
         comprehensive, quality care. Most of the work
         involves diabetes education.
   B. To the Public
      1. Our goal is to correct misconceptions and provide
         education regarding diabetes so that individuals may
         pursue a more normal, healthier lifestyle.
      2. We want to empower with information individuals
         who wish to take responsibility for management of
         their diabetes.
      3. We strive to alleviate development of predisposed
         complications and to provide early intervention.
      4. We provide comprehensive care.

Database Note

As with other diagnoses, the development and ongoing maintenance
of a database for the diabetes patients discharged from your hospital
can provide a targeted list of individuals who should be apprised of
ongoing education and screening events. Keep in mind that the more
education people have, the more likely they are to take responsibility
for their condition. The best service we can provide is to educate this
population.

SUMMARY

Diabetes is a condition with a large number of potential complications that patients bring into the continuum of care. Develop an understanding of the complications, study your patient population to identify the diabetes diagnosis, and determine which continuum components can be aggregated for promotional purposes. Educate physicians to use the continuum of care and develop mechanisms to ensure that physicians receive vital communications regarding the initial treatment and to facilitate the smooth return of patients. Within Chapter 20, "The Marketer's Toolbox," we have included samples of diabetes education flyers, along with case studies and grand rounds.

REFERENCES

1. American Diabetes Association 1989. Diabetes facts and figures.
2. American Diabetes Association 1989. Basic information series no. 15: Nerve complications—neuropathy.
3. American Diabetes Association 1989. Basic information series no. 11: Complications of diabetes.
4. American Diabetes Association 1989. Basic information series no. 16: Complications—impotence.
5. American Diabetes Association 1989. Basic information series no. 17: Heart and blood vessel complications.
6. American Diabetes Association 1989. Basic information series no. 14: Kidney complications (nephropathy).
7. American Diabetes Association 1989. Basic information series no. 12: Eye complications (retinopathy).

5

CHAPTER

Cardiac Services

According to the American Heart Association's publication, *Heart and Stroke Facts: 1997 Statistical Update* more than 57 million Americans have some form of cardiovascular disease.[1] Consider the association's diagnosis-specific numbers: coronary heart disease, 13.67 million; stroke, 3.89 million; high blood pressure, 50 million; and rheumatic heart disease, 1.38 million. It's hard to even imagine, isn't it? But given the prevalence of cardiovascular disease in the United States and with cardiac patients' predisposition to other conditions, providing a specialized continuum of care will become a necessity for hospitals. While many hospitals now provide quality care for the acute phase of the condition, hospitals that develop and implement an efficient continuum will benefit the patient, the community, and the financial goals of the facility. The American Heart Association reports that Americans will pay an estimated $259.1 billion in 1997 for CVD-related medical costs and disability. In order to implement the continuum of care successfully, we must move patients into and out of the system effectively. This will demand a new level of coordination within the facility and a new educational focus.

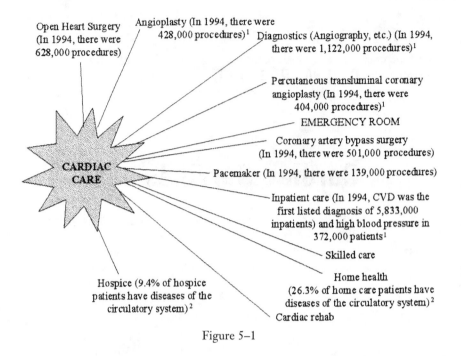

Open Heart Surgery
(In 1994, there were
628,000 procedures)

Angioplasty (In 1994, there were
428,000 procedures)[1] Diagnostics (Angiography, etc.) (In 1994,
there were 1,122,000 procedures)[1]

Percutaneous transluminal coronary
angioplasty (In 1994, there were
404,000 procedures)[1]

EMERGENCY ROOM

Coronary artery bypass surgery
(In 1994, there were 501,000 procedures)

Pacemaker (In 1994, there were 139,000 procedures)

Inpatient care (In 1994, CVD was the
first listed diagnosis of 5,833,000
inpatients) and high blood pressure in
372,000 patients[1]

Skilled care

CARDIAC
CARE

Hospice (9.4% of hospice
patients have diseases of the
circulatory system)[2]

Home health
(26.3% of home care patients have
diseases of the circulatory system)[2]

Cardiac rehab

Figure 5–1

Key components to system success are:

- Establishing a new approach to discharge planning to focus on planning the continuum and ensuring that the patient moves through the continuum to all appropriate levels of care
- Educating staff and physicians regarding the available continuum and patient eligibility
- Continually using the hospital's or system's internal management system information database to apprise potential patients of the continuum of services offered and how to access them
- Educating the community on the cardiac continuum of care and why it is important.

In considering who the target groups are for all of these services, it is easy to see that many of the diagnostic and acute care services are physician driven. The patient may be diagnosed in a physician's office as having high blood pressure and may be treated with medication. The physician will monitor the patient on an ongoing basis because he or she is at risk for a heart attack or stroke. The physician may suspect atherosclerosis, or hardening of the arteries, and begin to monitor levels of cholesterol and triglycerides in the bloodstream and to suggest lifestyle changes. This hypothetical patient may then present in the physician's office with complaints of angina (chest pain). Some patients may experience chest pain when they are exercising, walking, or feeling excited, because the blood supply to their heart is insufficient.

Angina can be treated with medication or surgical techniques to diagnose and to address the blood flow. Diagnostics have become important in our continuum of care, with facilities offering electrocardiograms and monitoring equipment. Cardiac catheterization is performed by injecting dye into the coronary arteries. This technique allows physicians to identify the blocked areas of the artery. When these areas are found, several procedures may address the blockage. Angioplasty is one such procedure; it is often referred to as *percutaneous transluminal coronary angioplasty*, or PTCA. More common is the term *balloon angioplasty*. A medical device is introduced into the artery, where it inflates like a balloon to widen the blocked area. This is not always successful, and sometimes the area does not stay clear. Another treatment is coronary artery bypass graft (CABG) surgery, in which physicians take a healthier piece of artery from another area and graft it into the place of the blocked area to restore blood flow. Conversely, the patient may suffer a heart attack in the emergency room or office with no history of heart problems. These patients can benefit during recovery from many different components of the continuum. Perhaps they will be treated in the skilled unit or discharged with home care services. In addition, PTCA or CABG (as well as heart attack) qualify them for cardiac rehab.

The American Heart Association's publication *Fact Sheet on Heart Attack, Stroke and Risk Factors* states that according to the Framingham Heart Study, an estimated 350,000 new cases of angina occur each year.[3] These patients may be routed into the organization's continuum as part of the diagnostic services. Of course, if a patient is in severe distress or suffers a heart attack—and the publication just mentioned states that "this year as many as 1.5 million Americans will have a new or recurrent heart attack"[3]—the entry to the continuum will be driven by location, reputation, or a combination of the two. In cardiac care, the goal is to have the public think of your facility's services first so that they consciously choose you. Given the emergency nature of a heart attack, this may not always occur. The challenge is to have such a cardiology continuum reputation established so that your postacute services are consciously chosen. In postacute care services, the referral process may be largely physician driven, but the influence of other referral sources is strong within this large population pool. The *Fact Sheet on Heart Attack and Stroke Risk Factors* states that "11,200,000 people alive today have a history of heart attack, angina pectoris (chest pain) or both." It is important to get to all levels of both influencers and decision makers to drive the referral process and ultimately to secure the choice of your facility as the healthcare provider.

   I. Target Groups
      A. Physicians
      B. Hospital-based employees
      C. General public
  II. Mechanisms
      A. Physicians
         1. Articles in medical staff newsletter
         2. One-to-one educational contacts
         3. Medical Director or program directors networking with physicians
         4. Physician office staff education
      B. Hospital-based employees
         1. Articles in hospital newsletter
         2. Payroll stuffers
         3. Seminars and in-service education
      C. General public
         1. Radio or television programs with physician experts
         2. Human interest stories in newspapers or senior publications with sidebars on diagnoses
         3. Screening events
            a. Blood pressure
            b. Cholesterol
            c. Fitness (may include percentage body fat, pulmonary screening, stress tests, etc.; can be as intensive as you choose within your legal counsel's constraints)
         4. Educational seminars (from informative to fun, education to cooking)

5. Public newsletters
6. Support groups
7. Business and industry groups
8. Direct mail
9. Billboards
10. Reporting on your research or internal studies
through the media
11. Health fairs

THE STRATEGY

Here our strategy is to establish the hospital as the provider of the cardiac continuum and to increase referrals to every step in the continuum of care:

- Physician specialists on the medical staff
- Emergency room
- Diagnostics
- Surgical services
- Telemetry unit or skilled unit
- Cardiac rehab
- Home care
- Hospice

DATABASE USE

Hospitals have at their disposal many information points that may be
virtually untapped in educating the public and generating referrals to
self-referral programs. One such program is outpatient cardiac rehabilitation. While admission to the program is by physician order, anyone can initiate a referral. Because of the fear associated with a cardiac
episode and the intense desire to "just go home," many individuals
may not be immediately interested in the continuum. However, continuum services may assist cardiac patients in taking responsibility for
their condition and changing their lifestyle.

Medicare is very specific regarding the eligibility requirement
for this program. The focus here is to attempt to assist those patients
who may be eligible but who have slipped out of the continuum of care
services loop. One method of facilitating education for this group is to

perform a quarterly search in the database for those patients within the Medicare diagnoses eligible for outpatient cardiac rehabilitation programs or ongoing seminars that the hospital may sponsor.

Once this is done, the next step may be an educational mailing to discuss the advantages of cardiac rehabilitation in assisting the patient to manage the cardiac condition, lessen recidivism, and so on. Most patients can benefit from reading an article from a medical journal that explains this approach to taking more control of their condition. Many patients erroneously believe that once the acute incident is over, they may return to their previous lifestyle. It is understandable that an individual's focus is discharge from the hospital, but our challenge as healthcare professionals is to assist patients in understanding the limitations of their conditions and the steps they may take to alter their lifestyles. Of course, this mailing would include a brochure regarding the continuum of cardiac care and information on how to access services.

Development of an ongoing database can facilitate mailings regarding upcoming screening events (cholesterol, blood pressure, etc.), support groups, and seminars that would be of benefit to the cardiac population.

SUMMARY

The cardiac patient population is both large and diverse, with individuals at varying levels of intensity and medical need. Our challenge is to establish our organizations as the premier providers with healthcare professionals and the public in order to attract patients to the continuum of care, whatever the level of need. While every community hospital cannot provide all of the needed interventions, each can offer particular components. Whatever you choose to do within the continuum, do it well. A sample coronary continuum of care brochure outline and program communications are included in Chapter 20, "The Marketer's Toolbox."

REFERENCES

1. American Heart Association 1997. Heart and stroke statistical update, pp. 3, 15, 27.
2. National Association for Home Care 1995. Basic statistics about home care, p. 5.
3. American Heart Association 1997. Fact sheet on heart attack, stroke and risk factors.

6

C H A P T E R

Neurology Services

In considering the promotion of neurology services, it is important to consider that many neurology diagnoses have a long product life cycle. Some individuals with diagnoses within this category will enter the acute care setting as trauma patients through the emergency room. These may include patients with spinal cord injuries with brain injuries, strokes and in coma. These types of patients will need both intensive and prolonged services at many levels within the continuum of care, some for a lifetime. The care will be focused on enhancing cognitive and physical status, with the goal of achieving the patients' maximum capabilities. Miraculous recoveries of these types of patients are often reported in print or television stories.

Within the category of neurological diagnoses we also see the more chronic patient. For example, chronic pain is defined as pain from injury or illness of at least six months duration. It affects millions of Americans and is perhaps one of the most misunderstood diagnoses that healthcare providers face. These patients may face medication dependency, loss of capabilities, loss of employment ability, and varying levels of frustration, anxiety, and depression. Depending on the condition of each patient, there may be benefit from surgical and/or medical intervention, as well as rehabilitation and vocational services within our continuums. Without a doubt it is one of the most complex areas to market, largely because of the level of understanding by the public and healthcare professionals. For far too many years, many if not all of these individuals were incorrectly labeled as malingerers rather than patients who required medical intervention. In many areas this old paradigm still exists, prompting us to search for creative methods to market services that are not well understood.

With other illnesses and conditions, this is often less of a problem. Persons with widely publicized neurological conditions such as Alzheimer's disease, may enter our system for initial diagnostics and then move through the system with continuing care. Many of these neurological conditions are progressive, with individuals requiring more services and support.

ALZHEIMER'S DISEASE

The diagnoses of high-profile Americans with Alzheimer's disease, such as former President Ronald Reagan, have increased knowledge of this condition. Today it is recognized as the most common cause of dementia, with approximately 10 percent of people over age 65 affected. The percentage rises to 47.2 percent for those age 85 or older.[1] The disease itself has no treatment, but some of the symptoms may be alleviated through medication. This progressive condition is the fourth leading cause of death in adults, after heart disease, cancer, and stroke.[2] As such, it must be included in our discussions on continuum. The individual may enter our continuum for diagnostic services—which may include laboratory and radiology tests, EEGs, CT scans, EKGs, neuropsychological testing, and a detailed medical history,[1] because there is no single test for Alzheimer's—and progressively move toward total care in the home or nursing home.

Consider the financial implications of Alzheimer's[1]:

- Alzheimer's is the third most expensive disease in the United States, after heart disease and cancer.
- The average lifetime cost per patient is $174,000, with a cost of $80 billion to $100 billion a year in the United States.
- More than seven of ten people with Alzheimer's live at home. Approximately 25 percent of their care is paid home care costing an average of $12,500 per year per patient.

- Half of all nursing home patients suffer from Alzheimer's or a related disorder. The average yearly cost for a patient's care in a nursing home is $42,000, but can exceed $70,000 in some areas of the country.

Alzheimer's patients may experience confusion, language problems, poor or impaired judgment, disorientation, and changes in personality. They eventually are totally unable to care for themselves.[1] The implications for our continuum of care components are significant to home care, assisted living, adult day care, long-term care, and hospice services. Many providers are meeting the challenges now. Long-term care facilities have developed Alzheimer's units with security systems for the safety of these patients. They emphasize cognitive status and quality of life. Local Alzheimer's chapters provide listings to families of long-term care facilities and other providers equipped to care for this special population. Many adult day care programs have focused entirely on participants with Alzheimer's and other memory problems. These programs also have security systems and focus on maintaining as much cognitive function as possible with special memory programs. Some have "wandering paths" so that these individuals may safely walk through an area with items to pick up and put down at will. Our challenge will be to enhance our components to meet the needs of this population and to prepare for the large numbers of Alzheimer's patients who will enter our continuum.

STROKE

Stroke could be viewed as a cardiovascular problem and addressed within the cardiology service section. However, we have chosen to include it in the neurology section because the brain is affected. Stroke and other neurological disorders bring our patients into the system often in emergency and diagnostic situations. The patient may undergo MRIs, CT scan, angiography, or other tests to determine carotid artery blockage and damage to the brain. According to the American Heart Association, "about 500,000 Americans suffer strokes each year. About 3,080,000 victims are alive today."[3] The product line, unfortunately, has a long life cycle because of the time required for recovery and the risk of successive strokes. A number of diagnostic and treatment services can be employed in the care of stroke patients (see Figure 6–1).

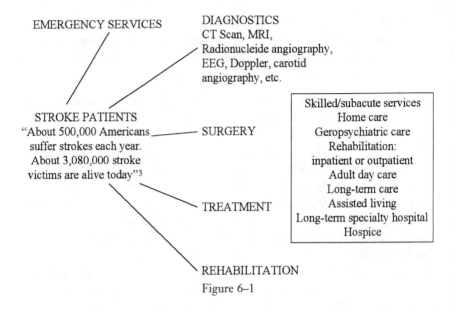

EMERGENCY SERVICES

DIAGNOSTICS
CT Scan, MRI,
Radionucleide angiography,
EEG, Doppler, carotid
angiography, etc.

STROKE PATIENTS
"About 500,000 Americans
suffer strokes each year.
About 3,080,000 stroke
victims are alive today"[3]

SURGERY

TREATMENT

REHABILITATION

Skilled/subacute services
Home care
Geropsychiatric care
Rehabilitation:
inpatient or outpatient
Adult day care
Long-term care
Assisted living
Long-term specialty hospital
Hospice

Figure 6–1

Surgery may be indicated. Medications can reduce the chance of clots and alleviate swelling in the brain. The stroke patient may be left with residual paralysis or weakness, cognitive difficulties (inability to think clearly and sequence thoughts), loss of sight, loss of hearing, or affected speech or swallowing. Consider these statistics from the American Heart Association:[4]

- Stroke is the third leading cause of death in the United States and a major cause of serious disability after diseases of the heart and cancer.
- The initial thirty-day case fatality for stroke is high, (averaging 38 percent); however, about 50 percent of those surviving the critical period are still alive seven years later.
- In the Framingham study, 31 percent of stroke survivors needed help in caring for themselves, 20 percent needed help walking, and 16 percent had to be institutionalized.

Given these facts, the development and promotion of the post-acute continuum for stroke patients will include rehabilitation services delivered inpatient, skilled, outpatient, or assisted living, adult day care, home care setting. Promotion of neurological services, both diagnostic and treatment, depend first upon having the appropriate specialty physicians on staff to deliver the care, equipment, and services to diagnose and successfully treat the individual, and second upon the successful tactics to promote them.

I. Target Groups
  A. Physicians
  B. Hospital-based employees
  C. General public
II. Mechanisms
  A. Physicians
    1. Articles in medical staff newsletter
    2. One-to-one educational contacts
    3. Medical director of specialty program networking with other physicians
    4. Physician office staff education
  B. Hospital-based employees
    1. Articles in hospital newsletter
    2. Continuum of care case studies at luncheons
    3. Payroll stuffers
  C. The general public
    1. Media—TV, radio, print
    2. Support groups
    3. Human interest stories
    4. Senior news vehicles
    5. Educational seminars
    6. Public newsletters
    7. Brochures in physicians' offices
    8. Health fairs
    9. Specialty programs, such as patient reunions

THE STRATEGY

The strategy is to establish your hospital as the neurology center in the area with a continuum of services, quality physicians, technology, and quality care, and to increase referrals at every step in the continuum of care, including the following:

- Emergency room
- Physician specialists

- Social workers and psychologists
- Diagnostics
- Surgical services
- Skilled nursing unit
- Rehab (inpatient and outpatient)
- Geropsychiatric (inpatient and outpatient)
- Home care
- Long-term care
- Adult day care

Also build a database to continually educate and inform individuals who may be at further risk. Some neurological conditions that may benefit from the continuum of care services are:

- Pain
- Back or neck surgery
- Degenerative disk disease
- Spinal injury
- Traumatic injury
- Tumor
- Guillain-Barré syndrome
- Neurologic disorders
- Multiple sclerosis
- Parkinson's disease
- Alzheimer's disease
- Brain injury
- Stroke

SUMMARY

Many areas within the diagnostic category of neurological conditions are often those with longer product life cycles. These patients will therefore often require medical intervention of some type on an ongoing basis. It is our mission to provide services that will meet their needs. Be aware of complementary services within your community and be prepared to direct patients appropriately to providers. We have included samples for program communications and public education on stroke in Chapter 20, "The Marketer's Toolbox."

REFERENCES

1. Alzheimer's Disease and Related Disorders Association, Inc. 1994. Alzheimer's disease: an overview.
2. Alzheimer's Disease and Related Disorders Association, Inc. 1994. Alzheimer's disease fact sheet.
3. American Heart Association 1996. Fact sheet on heart attack, stroke, and risk factors.
4. American Heart Association 1996. Heart and stroke facts.

TWO

INTERNAL STRATEGIES FOR THE CONTINUUM OF CARE

Strategically placing clients within current healthcare system pathways can be challenging. Because of the nature of the system and the complexity of the patient's needs and resources, patients, families, and healthcare professionals are often overwhelmed. The American healthcare system is changing drastically. The healthcare continuum has taken on new meaning for both patients and providers. This change is characterized by a much more dramatic emphasis on outcomes. This has been perhaps the greatest change in the field of healthcare. Is the change in American healthcare a positive change? Regardless of the answer, change is here.

In this section we focus on the internal issues of continuum placement, the analyses and the educational/marketing processes. Some marketing managers may judge some of these to be inapplicable to our focus. However, no promotional effort exists in a vacuum, and internal systems will either facilitate or thwart the continuum utilization process. This section will provide the big picture for the marketer and ways to assess the internal systems that affect referrals.

7

CHAPTER

Discharge Planning— Cross-Function, Not Cross-Purposes

Hospital-based discharge planning has evolved, with more changes to come. As the industry has developed clinical pathways and disease management protocols, the process of referrals and the departments responsible for them have changed dramatically (see Figure 7–1). As in other areas, it was the financial pressure from Medicare and managed care that drove the changes within the system.

In the past, social services representatives chiefly functioned to counsel patients and offer assistance in accessing community services. Later they completed applications for governmental programs such as Medicaid. As DRGs were implemented there was a new push for more proactive discharge planning. Suddenly, waiting for a bed to become available within the community was not such a good reason for holding up patient discharges. At this point many hospitals chose to employ nurses, in addition to social workers, for the discharge-planning process so discharges could be more proactively planned and coordinated clinically.

The evolution from discharge planning to case management was driven at least in part by specialty hospitals, such as rehabilitation and psychiatric facilities, that developed case-management departments as a way to market for commercial patients. These facilities sought to

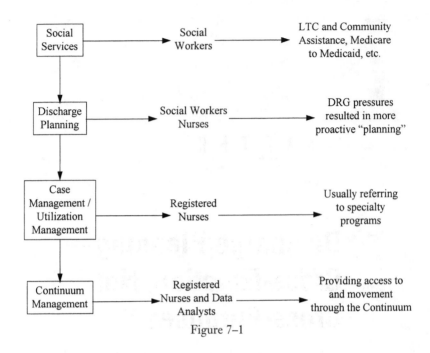

Figure 7–1

decrease their dependence on Medicare patients and increase the census of commercial payors who (at that time, in the 1980s) were considered by many to be better revenue sources than the Medicare patients. The presence of an efficient case-management system paved the way for specialty providers to actively market insurers, employers, private medical case managers, and third-party payors for the more lucrative patients (including a percentage of catastrophic injury patients) who were likely to have complex issues resulting in longer stays. Case managers focused on working successfully with insurance companies and other referral sources to streamline the delivery of care within stipulated guidelines or to advocate additional services for the patient. Communication and timely and accurate reports sent with the bill were the main foci of the case manager. Of course, within the communication function was the explicit expectation to generate more and more referrals. It is interesting to note, however, that as many of the specialty hospitals furloughed their social workers on "corporate directives," their stream of hospital-based referrals was often negatively affected for some time as their specialty social workers and the hospital-based social workers' peers commiserated.

The very system of peer relationships that they had diligently sought to encourage for referrals had indeed been successful.

With the growth of managed care edging out the more lucrative payor sources, provision and management of continuum services gains importance. Once again, to many facilities, Medicare may be a more attractive payor than some of the facilities' negotiated managed care contracts. Consider that many consultants advise that up to 35 percent of Medicare risk patient days can be ICU days, and that it is virtually impossible to shave days off the front of an admission. Continuum components are absolutely necessary to ensure the delivery of care within the most appropriate setting. Given this situation, registered nurses with experience as insurance case managers, knowledge of continuum criteria, a broad range of clinical expertise and access, and excellent physician and patient rapport appear to be the most qualified persons for this redesigned departmental function of case management. With these types of criteria, it is easy to see why many organizations build their "field of dreams" in continuum of care services but are disappointed by utilization statistics.

We believe that in the future many organizations will also include analysts within the department who will monitor all of the different managed care contracts (and their approved treatment settings and patterns), overlaying them with current patient stays and physician utilization and working closely with the RNs to expedite transfers to the most appropriate settings. If we assume that the right person is in the right position, we must then determine whether the tools exist to move the patients efficiently and whether the process can be supported at all levels within the organization.

TOOLS COMMONLY USED WITHIN THE CONTINUUM MANAGEMENT PROCESS

Discharge Rounds

These meetings are often unit based to discuss patients' discharges. Representatives of different programs often attend to identify appropriate patients.

Pro: They provide an opportunity to look at the total patient.

Con: The patient may be identified as suitable for several different programs; relationships and personalities within those programs may drive the referral process.

Census Sheet Screenings	Hospital specialty program representatives scan the morning census sheet by diagnosis. They may check charts and request a referral to evaluate patients from MDs or utilization management. *Pro:* Individuals most familiar with admission criteria are identifying appropriate patients. *Con:* Again, the same patient may appear suitable for multiple settings within the continuum, and the ultimate choice may not be made on appropriateness.
Chart Note/Flag	Hospital specialty program representatives or utilization management may affix "sticky notes" to charts identifying potential referrals after conducting an informal review of patients' charts. *Pro:* This may stimulate some thought by the referral source as to which site is appropriate. *Con:* The decision may be dictated by chance timing of a chart flag and made on a first come, first served basis. Chart notes may identify patients for a given program but be insufficient to educate the physician on what makes individuals qualify for one service over another.
Daily Outlier/Cost Printout	Some hospitals generate a daily report on each patient's stay and the associated costs. Many systems providing such a report are managing the care closely so that every day's stay and associated costs can be monitored and continuum entry is facilitated.

The utilization management process is the single most valuable tool for hospitals in developing a continuum focus. However, most facilities view this as an event (discharge by discharge) and not a process (continuum entry).

It will take time and resources to perfect this process. But consider that some hospitals are willing to direct tens of thousands of dollars (and even more) into advertising campaigns for visibility while they are unwilling to determine how better to serve patients within their systems. As anyone in sales can attest, it is much more cost-effective to maintain a customer (patient) relationship than to develop new ones. While advertising for the purpose of attracting new patients will be an ongoing process, facility managers may see the necessity for extravagant expenditures in this area lessen if the facility can become continuum-driven. This ultimately benefits both the individual and the community as a whole.

However, this process is much more difficult than developing a new advertising campaign because it involves change. The focus must shift from a single function to a cross function that will at first divide teams. Specialty hospitals experienced this years ago in restructuring departments, moving from social work to case management. This process requires ongoing monitoring of systems. It may seem at first unnecessary and cumbersome to those both preparing and reviewing the reports but in time will yield a return on the investment.

Facilities successful in continuum management are providing cost-effective, quality care by moving patients into less intense settings and are using this to market to managed care organizations. This will be detailed more in Chapter 18 on insurers and continuum services.

STRATEGIC ANALYSIS AND THE PLANNING PROCESS

The first step in assessing the current process against the desired process is conducting a situation analysis. This involves objectively scrutinizing the systems in place and then determining how future monitoring will occur.

Situation Analysis

Current Process	Eventual/Desired
Length-of-stay emphasis with a single discharge focus	Focus on the continuum
Programs or services may drive the process according to their budgets with a departmental rather than a big-picture focus. In addition, downsizing or re-structuring within an organization may fuel program managers' or representatives' drive for census building for their own job security. This may also be a concern for staffing patterns and professionals on the unit who do not wish to rotate work on other units.	Patient's best interests at heart

Current Process	Eventual/Desired
Contract-managed units may/may not be continuum focused. Many facilities choose to use contract-management companies because they have expertise in specialty areas and because the facility management believes that the contract-management group will build census. If the continuum focus is not shared with the management group or the group feels intense pressure to build census, the best interests of the continuum and patient may be compromised. There should be shared responsibility for the success of all hospital continuum services.	Contract-managed units as part of the continuum with big-picture focus
Employees uneducated on programs	Employees advocate and actively promote the continuum to patients
Physicians knowledgeable about DRGs	Physicians knowledgeable and supportive of the continuum concept

We recommend a continuum analysis to determine where a hospital or system is in the development of continuum management. This is a two-step process, as follows:

1. Identification of current processes in place for routing patients

   - Who participates
   - Process efficiency
   - How quickly patients are moved after referral
   - Program or continuum focus
   - Preadmission programs in place
   - Preadmission programs that could be developed
   - Main driver of the process—physicians or utilization management (UM)

CASE STUDY

A hospital had recently opened a new skilled unit and was disappointed in the ramp-up of the program. Our investigations found that before opening the unit, representatives from the skilled facility across the street had participated in the hospital's discharge planning rounds and developed good relationships with department personnel. They continued to sit in at the meetings and were good at educating the discharge planners about why a patient was better served in their skilled unit.

CASE STUDY

I visited a small hospital with two RN discharge planners to evaluate their process for routing patients into their new skilled nursing unit. (The census ramp-up was slower than expected, given the acute care census.) The analysis began with a review of all of the discharge face sheets for the past year to the present year to date. It was easy to see that many patients were sent outside of the hospital for skilled services instead of to the new unit. After a thorough review of all sheets for diagnoses, physician patterns, and so on, I met with the two nurses. After reviewing the findings, I asked why so many patients appropriate for skilled care were being sent to other providers in the area. Imagine my surprise when they said, "Well, we send them out because there is just so much paperwork (admission and discharge) when we move them into the unit here, and when we call one of the freestanding facilities, they take care of everything."

I then met with the chief financial officer (CFO) of the hospital (the department reported up to the CFO) and he indicated he didn't have adequate time to review the type of monthly reports that we were suggesting. (An interesting footnote: He is no longer in that position.)

2. Data Analysis

- Reviewing discharge planning logbooks or records: What were the discharge patterns for the past year (total discharges and the discharges to different settings for percentages)?
- All external referrals: What reason was listed for external referrals to programs competing with the same type of existing hospital-based program? Are there any patterns within these external referrals (reasons, physician, UM representative, location, specialty services, etc.)? What percentage of patients were referred out of the system?

With this information and objective recommendations provided by the data, facilities may begin the reengineering and strategic planning processer to determine where they have service gaps and opportunities to fill the unmet needs of the community. Ideally, this information will provide optimal insight when overlaid with an analysis that includes the following:

- Review of Management Information Systems printouts for DRGs by physician, payor, and length of stay
- Referral and admissions analysis for every specialty program
- Study, by each specialty program, of information on patients referred—e.g., admissions vs. nonadmissions (conversion rates), reasons for nonadmissions, diagnosis, physicians, etc.
- Referrals from specialty programs to other continuum services

This information can provide the hospital system with knowledge of where the process is or is not working and can facilitate the redesign of organizational systems. It can be the single most important tool in meeting hospital or system continuum of care goals.

CREATING ACCOUNTABILITY AND IDENTIFYING OPPORTUNITIES

We recommend maintaining a discharge logbook and filing the fact sheets of the discharged patients with any handwritten notes. Each month a report should be sent to the chief executive officer, chief financial officer, and chief operating officer and should include the following:

- Number of patients processed through the UM/continuum management department
- Number of referrals to hospital/system services
- Number of referrals to external services by category with rationale
- Cross-reference with specialty program reports.

For incorporation into this report, we suggest discharge logs be reviewed from specialty programs and monthly statistics provided to attach to the UM report. Statistics should include the following:

- Number of patients referred
- Number of patients admitted
- Conversion rate (percent of patients referred to those admitted)
- Specifics on patients referred by UM, and if not admitted, why not
- Patients (not admitted to program or those discharged) referred to continuum services

CASE STUDY

A hospital administrator was perplexed that the acute rehab unit was not as full as hospital projections suggested that it would be. After conducting due diligence, she learned that patients were leaving the system for other programs in town. She notified the discharge planning department that if patients who qualified for rehabilitation chose another provider, she wanted the discharge planner to come to her office to personally explain the choices. She learned about perceptions of her unit as compared with the competition. Soon she was able to address issues that could be improved, and to identify areas of misconception regarding the unit on the part of the physician staff. Soon more physicians were educated regarding the capabilities of the unit and more patients began to choose to remain at her facility. (The moral of the story is: What you don't know about perceptions can hinder your success.)

SUMMARY

As marketers prepare to meet the challenges of continuum promotion, they must first turn their efforts inward to analyze the current continuum referral flow. At times, they will proactively function as internal change agents, questioning current practices. To become successful, they must understand the internal process and its implications to the marketing effort. It will not be easy and will involve the political hazards of crossing organizational lines. Maintain focus on the organization's financial goals. The final product will be not only a more efficient organization but also a more effective marketing professional, well equipped to assume more responsibility within the management team.

8 CHAPTER

Evaluating the Efficiency of the Intake Process

It all starts innocuously enough with a phone call or a walk-in, but sometimes it can go very, very wrong. Some managers never stop to think how much revenue and how many clients are lost to other facilities before we even consider them as potential patients.

THE INQUIRY PROCESS

Do you really know what happens when the phone rings? How many rings does it take before it is answered? How many times can one human being possibly be transferred after being on seemingly endless hold? It is a good idea to call your programs at odd hours to test the system and determine if the system is user-friendly.

What is the programmatic educational level of your first-line contacts? Are they treated as valuable team members and invited to department meetings, or are there barriers in providing the necessary information to make them and the program more successful? As a colleague of mine says, we often take the person in the facility who is paid the least and knows the least about the program and identify them as the first-line contact. Whether this is the receptionist or the ward clerk, we have seen some creative ways to address the problem. We recommend that everyone focus on helping these people and teaching them more about the program. Sitting with them, helping them on tours, and providing opportunities to learn are the best ways to educate them in the program. Have they shadowed a direct care provider or a patient to actually know what happens in the program? We advocate providing a fact book about the program. It has individual sheets about every aspect of the program, about who appropriate patients are and how they may benefit, and about rudimentary payor coverage so that the first-line contacts have a resource at their fingertips. Consider that these individuals make the first impression of the program. If they don't know answers to questions, your facility may not sound like a place the prospective patient should go.

CASE STUDY

Recently I phoned a skilled facility in the South as part of a competitive assessment. The phone rang twice and was answered professionally. I inquired about the facility and was given concise directions. I explained that I was looking for a facility that could provide care for my family member who had experienced a stroke and asked if the facility accepted patients with that type of illness. (Most nursing facilities with Medicare units welcome this type of patient.) Imagine my surprise when I was told, "I don't know, hold on." After being on hold seemingly forever (and if I were truly a family member I would have hung up!), the individual returned and said, "Yes, we do." She volunteered no more information and did not ask me for any information, nor did she ask me to come by to tour or speak with anyone. Another referral lost.

CASE STUDY

I traveled to a Gulf Coast city and made plans to tour five facilities within a fifty-mile radius. I phoned all of the facilities to get directions. When I phoned one of the facilities I explained that I was from out of town and would be by to tour that day. The receptionist was quite alarmed and asked if I had spoken with a representative in admissions. I stated that I had not. She then asked if I could come by the following day when the admissions coordinator would be back. I again stated that I was in from out of town and needed to come that day. At this point she said, "Well, don't come until this afternoon and maybe she'll be here." With all of the competition these days, I was quite surprised that anyone could afford to hesitate on responding to referrals and wondered if the management had ever conducted mystery shopping calls themselves.

Do you really know your inquiry process internally? Are you absolutely confident of its efficiency? Read through the following self-assessment and consider developing one for the next meeting within your organization.

Intake System Self-Assessment

What happens if the phone line(s) are busy?

Do you know who accepts inquiry calls for your specialty program on:

All three shifts?

Afternoon/evenings?

Weekends and holidays?

Is the receptionist educated in how to respond to basic and specific questions (can she respond without referring the caller to someone else)?

Are inquiry forms centrally located?

Are the calls or walk-ins recorded on an inquiry form?

Is the form routed to facilitate the referral?

Is the offer made to have a program representative phone? Does this occur?

Is the offer made to arrange a tour with transportation if needed?

Do you know what is the percentage of referrals from inquiries in your program(s)?

Do you know what is the percentage of admissions from referrals in your program(s)?

Do you know if there are any trends in inquiries or referrals by month?

Do you know what is the percentage of referrals from your program(s) routed elsewhere within the continuum?

INQUIRY TIPS

We offer the following inquiry tips:

- Every inquiry should have a form filled out to record the call. These can be individually developed for every program, with specific details as needed. The inquiry forms (see the Worksheets on pages 69,

70, and 71) or a book of them, organized in a three-ring binder, should be kept in a central place or several places so that anyone can pick them up and walk through an inquiry when a call comes in. Keeping the inquiry forms in several areas also prevents inquiries being taken on scraps of paper and later lost. A person may be designated to collect the inquiry forms daily throughout the entire organization.

- Gather all possible information. Listen and ask questions. Sometimes you can repeat some points for your own clarification, to get more details, and to show that you are listening, but don't be a parrot. The individuals who are taking inquiries could most likely benefit from sales training because these techniques are sales by phone. If you can't provide training because of resource allocation, buy a couple of books or head to the library and have sessions from the books. Again, there is always a creative way to educate your staff.

Although the inquiry form needs to be complete, you should focus on the client, not the paper. Recently on one of my mystery shopping trips, the intake coordinator spent more time on the paperwork than she did "taking my temperature" regarding the referral or on the tour. The coordinator was trying to obtain information to complete all the admission paperwork and even asked for copies of Medicare and insurance cards, even though I candidly stated that I was just trying to narrow down the number of providers. Unfortunately, I would have selected another provider who was more interested in my mother than in the paperwork. This can be a delicate balancing act if the inquiry is taken in person. Ask if you can take some notes, but don't look like a stenographer. You should be able to add much more to the sheet after a comfortable conversation together is finished and the visitor has left.

- Provide directions as necessary. You would be shocked to learn how many people couldn't find their way out of a paper bag with an atlas. Keep directions with maps in the inquiry book. Make certain that the sets of directions are from all possible major highways. Nothing looks more foolish than an employee who can't tell you how to get to where he or she works. There is a subtle message here that reflects on the facility. In addition, if it doesn't sound easy (presentation, presentation, presentation) I am probably not going. Make it easy for me to choose you. When I schedule an appointment, offer to send me directions that include a map.

- Route as soon as possible to the appropriate person. Often an inquiry conversation ends with the phrase, "and someone will call you

INQUIRY FORM

Caller name: _____ Date: _____

Address: _____ Time: _____

Phone number: _____ Call received by: _____

Nature of the call: _____

_____

_____

Re: (name of potential patient, relationship) _____

    Cardiac rehab   ❐   Assisted living   ❐

    Long-term care   ❐   Geropsych (day)   ❐

    Adult day care   ❐   Rehab (inpt)   ❐

    Home health   ❐   Rehab (outpt)   ❐

    Geropsych (inpt)   ❐   Other _____

How did you hear about this service: _____

Routed to: _____ for Follow-up _____

Outcome: _____

Scheduled   Admitted   Did not admit   (Circle one)   Date: _____

Other/Why   Specify: _____

INQUIRY INFORMATION

Caller's name: _____ Ph # (day/eve) _____

Relation to prospect:_____ Date: _____ Time: _____

Prospect: _____ Sex _____ Age _____

Current location _____ Phone _____

Date admission desired _____

Diagnosis/Condition: _____

Physician _____ Phone _____

Resp. party: Same as caller? _____ If no, name _____

Relation to prospect _____

Phone (day/eve) _____/_____ Send brochure? _____

Room: Priv Semi-Priv   Stay: Long term   Short term   Respite ____

Notes: _____

_____

_____

_____

Referred from (hosp, friend, church, etc) _____

Tour information: Given _____ Time _____Outcome _____

                          _____

Follow-up calls: _____

Date _____   Comments _____

                          _____

Date _____   Comments _____

                          _____

Date _____   Comments _____

                          _____

FINAL OUTCOME: _____

_____

_____

HOSPITALIZED RESIDENTS:

Prospect's status prior to hospitalization: _____

_____

Dates/types of surgeries _____

NOTES: _____

_____

CONDITIONS AND CARE NEEDS

CURRENT STATUS (circle or fill in the blank)

GENERAL INFORMATION

Height _____ Weight _____

ADL SKILLS   **(max/min)**   **(max/min)**

Self-care   Bathing assist   Dressing assist   Total assist

Ambulatory status

Ambulatory   Assist w/amb   Assist w/trans   Nonamb   Wheelchair

Bedridden   Walker/cane/other _____ Freq of falls _____

ELIMINATION STATUS

No assist   Assist to/from   Bedside commode   Total assist

Incont of bowel: rarely   occasional (1/week)   frequent   total

Incont of bladder: rarely   occas   freq   tot   catheter   diapers

SKIN STATUS

Normal   Dry   Decubitus   Other   Describe (if necessary) _____

_____ Treatments/Dressings _____

NUTRITIONAL STATUS

No assist   Assist w/meals   Feeder   Tube feeder(NG/G)

Special diet _____ Supplements _____

MENTAL AND BEHAVIORAL STATUS

General info: _____

Alert   Oriented   Forgetful   Confused   Lethargic

Passive   Cooperative   Uncooperative   Combative   Smoker

Wanders (how often, etc) _____ Problems: _____

_____

COMMUNICATION AND SENSORY SKILLS

Vision: _____

Hearing: _____

Speech: _____

MEDICATION AND OTHER INFO

Medications _____

Other _____

back," but somehow they never do. Tell me exactly who will call and make certain that they do. Again, a formal inquiry form with notations for follow-up will help greatly.

■ Respond in a timely fashion. If you do not respond quickly, your competitor probably already has.

■ Provide tracking information so that it may be analyzed or analyze it yourself. Are there any patterns to those persons who do not convert to patients? Is it location, lack of transportation, one payor with whom there is no agreement with, or another pattern?

■ Remember that inquiries are potential patients or community members who need the organization as a resource. Apply the Golden Rule and treat them as you would want to be treated.

THE IMPORTANCE OF TOURS

If a picture is worth a thousand words, then surely a tour is the key to census. Unfortunately, many of us do not focus on tours. The following are some ideas about conducting successful tours:

■ Know your facility or program and believe you can sell it. Half the battle is knowing the features and benefits so that you can emphasize the ones that the potential customer is interested in. Having a thorough knowledge of the product is half the battle. Knowledge begets confidence that you are prepared for the tour or the inquiry. Believing that you can sell the program is the other half. Often, you don't even need to know everything about a program if you truly believe in it and can tell why it is important to receive treatment or services. Once you have seen the results of a program and how it can change the life of an individual, you can be a believer—which is why we recommend shadowing patients to learn more about programs and services.

■ Prepare. Leave nothing to chance. When you arrive in the facility daily, walk around to check on the status of housekeeping and other departments. Are they presentable? Turn on the lights everywhere so that the building looks like there are patients there and it is bright and welcoming. Turn on the overhead sound system so there is a relaxing ambiance. (Choose the station for the customers, not the staff.) Determine if there should be an overhead announcement code for tours or if an employee will go through ahead of the tour to check details.

■ Know your patients, clients, families, and all employees. One contributor related that one day he was giving a tour to a prospective admission and spoke to a new employee. Unfortunately, he called the employee by the wrong name. The employee became very upset and pointed out his mistake loudly with additional comments. He apologized and continued his tour. He revisited this employee and again apologized. Consider the impressions we leave upon our visitors.

It is beneficial to have solid knowledge of the employees, clients, residents, and patients so you can "read" them. If someone is having a bad day and it shows on their face, introduce someone else.

Knowing everyone and having the ability to call individuals by name is a strong statement regarding programs. In healthcare, we are a caring business. However, during a tour many people forget this. Generally we would speak to everyone we pass while in the facility, but suddenly we are conducting a tour and have tunnel vision. We become so focused on the tour (the task at hand) that we exclude everything else from interfering. Our staff, caring and friendly, knows we are "on a tour" and if they recognize the importance of tours (after hearing this repeatedly) may even unconsciously move to one side of the hall and not speak to us during a tour. The message that is unwittingly given is that we are not a friendly organization. Staff should be inserviced upon joining the organization regarding the benefits of tours and their own role in the success of tours. (Refer to Chapter 16 on videos in assisted living for incorporating this into the orientation.) Introduce any people who have agreed to recommend the facility. At this point you can walk away and let the conversation occur and return in a few minutes. Let your customers sell your services for you.

■ Be knowledgeable regarding regulations and financial coverages. There is no need to discuss the intricacies of financial coverage in many cases. But your representatives should know the basics of Medicare coverage (Part A and Part B) and the utilization process or verification as related to insurance. Many times as our associates have gone on mystery shopping tours of facilities, they have "decided" on the provider whose staff demonstrated a knowledge of coverage or provided booklets regarding it. You can instruct your staff members conducting tours on weekends, holidays, and evenings to direct attention to the booklet and assure the individual touring that a follow-up call from the correct team member will discuss this in depth.

▪ Reconsider just how "casual" casual day is. This is healthcare, not retail. The appearance of the physical plant and the staff is the only way 99 percent of the public develops their judgment on quality care. We recognize that casual day is a way to build morale with the staff, but consider how far you want to go. Some facilities prohibit jeans or shirts with no collars, T-shirts with slogans, and so on. If you are committed to casual days, consider having a sign made for the entrance that says, "Every (day of the week) we observe casual day." At least in this way, visitors will not assume that this is the usual state of professionalism at your facility.

▪ Enforce the uniform/dress code. Again, this relates to the public's perception of the quality of care delivered within. In many skilled and assisted living facilities and long-term care settings, providers rebelled against uniforms with the rationale that "its their home, not a hospital." Unfortunately, this approach has cost many organizations census. Perception is everything. Some facilities have returned to uniforms and lab jackets for healthcare professionals. Recently, we toured a skilled unit where the nurses all wore their caps. When we asked the director of nursing about this she replied that the older generation had a certain perception regarding nurses. Management had consciously decided to require the caps so that the older people would not only feel more comfortable but would know which staff members were nurses.

▪ Use props, especially if there will be high traffic during an event. Picture boards, photographs of different staff and departments, calendars, activity schedules, thank you letters and cards, awards, and recognitions are excellent props for our tours. We have seen this done effectively with banners that said, "Congratulate us on our recent accreditation," or "Another deficiency free survey!" Professional staff may frame continuing education certificates. If you don't blow your own horn, no one else will. If you are sponsoring an event such as an open house and traffic will be flowing, sometimes without tour guides, staff different stations with an expert in the field or use large posters to describe the equipment or area and why it is important.

▪ Sell what you have. There are, no doubt, things you would change about your program or physical plant if you could. Maybe it would be location, maybe the color scheme or the carpet. Sell what you have and believe in it. Perhaps the most incredible story I have heard about this is related to a long-term care facility in the South.

The facility has a large number of three-bed rooms (wards). Although there are competitors with newer, nicer facilities, this facility stays full. It seems the administrator conducts all of the tours and tells families that with three residents in the rooms, more staff members are in and out and they will more than likely receive even more attention than if they were in a private room. There is a silver lining to every cloud!

■ Don't be penny-wise and pound-foolish with marketing: Don't focus on new brochures and promotional materials to the detriment of other areas. As one contributor put it, "Housekeeping counts, as do the little touches of decorations and flowers." He says a coat of paint is "marketing" just as much as an ad is. Look at your areas closely. Do they promote your programs?

CASE STUDY

A hospital recently opened a new outpatient program. The staff concentrated on marketing and getting the word out that they had opened. Equipment had been purchased and appropriate staff employed. Unfortunately, the lobby of the new area was empty save the old chairs had been placed in the area from storage.

■ Share personal experience and knowledge: If you or someone you are close to has experienced this type of care, share it. Empathy is powerful.

■ If the unthinkable happens, control your reaction, but get angrier than they do: If something unfortunate happens right in front of you, address it immediately. Show your concern in a measured way. Control your response to criticisms—they are inevitable because many people have misconceptions regarding health care. Don't ignore misconceptions, even if the patient in question is inappropriate for your program. Remember, this is your only opportunity as a provider to modify or replace old paradigms or to address deliberate misinformation given by competitors.

■ Respond to current clients: Again, many of us on tours are so focused on the immediate task at hand that we forget our jobs as healthcare providers. Remember that actions speak louder than words.

CASE STUDIES

During the best tour I have ever been on, the clinician kept excusing herself to respond to those who needed or asked for some type of assistance. I knew without a doubt that this person was caring and that this organization provided good care. (Yes, I know, there are pessimists among you who think this implied a lack of staff, but this person focused on the current customers and in doing so sold me.)

In the best example of what *not* to do on a tour, I can share what I saw recently in Florida. An individual in a wheelchair stopped as we approached, gestured and looked down the hall. I speak no Spanish, but it was very apparent to me that this person was asking the clinician that I was with to help her down the hall. The clinician conducting my tour responded, "I don't speak Spanish" and walked away.

■ Manage expectations: During a tour you can "take a temperature" to learn about prospective clients' expectations regarding such issues as the type of care that will be provided. This is your chance to gently guide expectations. If you can proactively address issues and prepare an individual for admission to your program, you can possibly head off misconceptions and issues that may arise during treatments. You can work smarter, not harder, to alleviate complaints and problems. Correspondingly, don't make promises that the organization cannot fulfill. Some individuals get so involved in the sale that they will promise almost anything to get the admission. Resulting difficulties often surface during the treatment. Staff members should realize that they cannot meet every stated need and some individuals will be better served by other programs. This situation often exists between sales and production, or in our industry, between marketing and operations.

■ Provide Tour Education to Your Staff: Everyone in the building should be prepared to conduct tours, with nights and weekend also covered by a protocol. We recommend that you develop and implement tour training for your facility and include inquiry protocols. One of our contributors provided the following tour script for a long-term care hospital:

> "Hello, Mr./Mrs./Ms. _____ my name is _____ and I am (mention your job). We welcome the opportunity to give you a tour of our facility. On the left of the reception area are the adminis-

trative offices. You can see from these framed certificates that we are accredited by JCAHO and CARF (explain these). Behind the reception area is the admissions coordinator's office. She will assist your family member with his/her admission to our hospital. If you have any questions or concerns, other than what I can help you with, you may reach her between 8 A.M. and 5 P.M., Monday through Friday. Our nurse liaison will also be glad to assist. Please feel free during your patient's stay with us to bring any questions or concerns to the attention of the admissions coordinator, social worker, director of nursing, director of therapy, marketing director, administrator, or any staff member.

On your right is one of our conference areas. Our dining room is here on the left, and we encourage all our patients, as they are able, to enjoy their meals here rather than in their rooms. The scenic view is very popular with our patients and their families, who often come in to relax. Guests are welcome for meals. If you would like to purchase a meal ticket ($3), you may do so through the receptionist/phone operator. We do ask that you let us know a few hours before mealtime, or the night before if it is for breakfast.

Adjoining the dining room is our therapeutic recreation room. Our specialist provides many opportunities for patients to enjoy activities such as painting, woodworking, needlework, puzzles, barbecues, and board games, and also invites in guest performers. We have pet therapy, which our patients enjoy very much. Often our patients enjoy outings in our hospital van assisted by therapists and other staff members. We have three separate wings in our hospital. Right now we are in the north wing. (Ask what room is available to show the guests.) You will notice that there is a television, telephone, and closet for each patient. The beds are electronic, each with a call light. (Open closets and the bathroom door. Turn lights on. Pull up or open blinds to display the view. Point out that every room has a view.) Depending on availability, we offer semiprivate and private rooms. Occasionally, a patient requesting a private room may have to admit into a semiprivate room and then move as a private room becomes available.

We encourage our patients to bring a few small personal items from home, such as photos, a plant, or a favorite afghan to make their stay more comfortable.

This is our east wing. We place our patients in each wing according to their level of independence and medical needs. As you can see, there is a scenic view from these rooms, as well. The office of our medical director, Dr. _____, is at the end of this hall. Either he or one of our other staff physicians will meet with your family member daily, to assess his/her needs. The admitting physician will assist the team in planning goals. We will schedule an appointment with his/her family doctor upon discharge.

(As you walk to and board the front elevator, mention team conference.) Every other week, our team of therapists, nurses, attending physician, dietitian, pharmacist, case manager, and social worker meet to set and review goals and objectives to improve the functional abilities of your family member. They also discuss the discharge plan, which the nurse liaison can discuss with you initially.

(Exiting the elevator on the ground floor, point out but do not walk to the social work/case management area. Show the speech therapy area, the team conference room, and orientation meeting room. Mention the beauty/barber shop across from the meeting room. Show a patient room in the south wing, and then point out the whirlpool area [mention one in each wing] and the respiratory therapy area, with its close proximity to the pulmonary wing, the east wing, point out that there are piped in gases set up in each room in this wing.)

(Walk to the left down the middle hall, walking north.) To our right is a snack room for staff and family and visitors. (Open the door and show the vending machines.) We also have a microwave and refrigerator that you are welcome to use. (Continue past the elevator, pointing out the second elevator, and show the pharmacy on the left.) A licensed pharmacist on staff prepares medications. (Show the activity of the daily living room on the left. You may need a key.) In this room, our patients practice and retrain the skills that they will need to regain as much independence as possible. In our kitchen and bathroom, our patients can learn to use adaptive equipment and safety techniques and find ways to conserve energy with the supervision of our therapists.

Our next room on the left is where our therapists do their planning and charting. In close proximity is our spacious gym. The expansive view creates a very enjoyable atmosphere that promotes the well-being of our patients. As you look out beyond, you can see a wheelchair accessible ramp that winds around reflection pools and a gazebo. Patients and families are encouraged to use this area. On special occasions, you may see patients having barbecues or parties out here.

(Walk to the pain management center.) This is the pain management center. It has state-of-the-art equipment and is staffed by physicians who perform procedures to alleviate chronic pain. As you see, there is a separate entrance, and it is closely connected to the gym area. It is very convenient for the patients. We treat patients on an outpatient basis as well as inpatient. (If the center is unlocked, enter and ask the secretary if you may tour the back patient area.) There are four patient rooms on the left, an x-ray procedure room in the back with a c-arm, where fluoroscopy can be performed. A waiting area on the right is for pre- and postprocedures, as needed.

(Walk back to the elevator at the front of the building, so that you exit the elevator in the lobby.) Are there any other questions that I might help you with? I may not have the answers, but I will be happy to get them for you.

As you can see, we have a lot to offer. I know that our staff will try in every way to make this an excellent stay for your family member. While we have twenty-four-hour nursing care and therapy six days a week, we work hard to make this feel less like a hospital and more like home, as much as possible. We encourage our patients to wear their own clothes. Usually loose-fitting casual clothes with tennis shoes work well. (At this point, return the keys to the receptionist and ask for brochures for the visitors. These should have the admissions co-ordinator's card in the slots. Walk the guests to the front door and tell them you'll look forward to welcoming their family member. Thank them for their visit.)

■ Develop a Tour Checklist for Educational Purposes: The following checklist may be helpful until the process becomes natural.

Tour Checklist Did you first stop to listen to what the individual had to say regarding:

- the prospective resident/patient/client?
- their own personal objections to overcome?
- the diagnosis or condition?
- the services they expressed a need for?
- their payor source?
- the timeline for a decision or immediacy of need?
- the decision makers involved?

Had you checked all areas for readiness before the tour?

- All areas clean and open, or are keys available?
- If your facility has a protocol of overhead tour announce-ment (paging) or having a staff member go ahead, did you follow it?
- During the tour, did you visit only the appropriate areas?

As you conducted the tour did you

- speak to all those clients, patients, employees, and visitors that you encountered?
- respond to call lights and requests or ask another staff member to do so?
- pick up any trash off the floor? (and not just step around it)
- discuss the items as indicated during tour-education sessions?

SUMMARY

Many people do not realize that improving tours and inquiries is one way to effect your marketing system immediately. It is much more costly to generate additional inquiries and referrals than to convert the appropriate ones that you have already generated. One assisted living organization conducts tour education and then "bonuses" the employee who closes a sale via the tour. We encourage you to conduct an inspection of your organization's approach to inquiries and tours and believe you just may discover some revenue-recovery opportunities.

9

CHAPTER

Analyzing Acute Care Discharges and Conversion Rates for Planning Purposes

Most hospitals have a great deal of information at their disposal. However, not all facilities or systems fully use this information. We encourage you to investigate the reports generated through your facility's management information system department and apply their use every day in managing patient flow through the continuum of care.

Hospital DRG runs can be sorted many different ways to tell you more about the practice profiles of the medical staff. One way is sorting to determine the payer mix of patients discharged by physicians and review the types of patients seen. Of assistance to both the utilization review (UR) department and program marketers is length of stay (LOS) information and admission trends by month. Other possible sorts are as follows:

Potential Sorts and Possible Information

Commercial/managed care discharges (by payor)

Types of patients

LOS by payor

Practice profile

Opportunities to contract for entire continuum

Medicare discharges by DRG by physician

Practice profile

Average length of stay (ALOS)

ALOS vs. national, state, or budgeted ALOS

Loss per case

Educational needs of individual

Physicians and medical staff

Note the educational needs of individual physicians and the medical staff. Although many people expect physicians to be aware of Medicare regulations, billing, and admissions criteria, the fact is that many physicians are uncertain of how to access some of the continuum services, and may have some misconceptions regarding them. This is often a factor in new skilled/subacute units because some physicians may perceive the units to be "nursing homes" inside the hospital and must be educated regarding the skill level of staff and appropriate patients for the unit. Another common situation is with acute rehab units. Some physicians may focus so closely on strokes (a common admission diagnosis) that they do not consider other diagnostic categories to benefit patients who have experienced a decline in function. Additionally, many new geropsych programs, both inpatient and outpatient, have experienced disappointing census ramp-ups because of misconceptions and a lack of pre-opening education.

Using such printouts will facilitate a targeted effort (by multiple hospital-based professionals) in assisting physicians with appropriate access to the continuum.

OVERLAYING SPECIALTY UNIT/PROGRAM ADMISSIONS

Every specialty unit or program will generally keep a manual or computerized logbook of admissions. Units and programs that are marketing their services will also maintain a logbook or file on referrals to compare to admissions. The information maintained is often inconsistent and may not be as complete as is necessary for marketing purposes. We have been asked to analyze facility information only to learn that all the inquiry sheets were discarded if the patient was not admitted! In effect, the most important information to the program was unavailable. Implementing policies and procedures to maintain records for referrals and admissions can be invaluable to facilities. A few samples follow. Most facilities have similar forms because there are only so many pertinent items to record.

SAMPLE POLICIES AND PROCEDURES

Policy

It will be the policy of the program to establish or augment the existing method of recording referral and admissions data for the compilation of statistical data.

Procedure

Patient information will be collected from the time of initial referral to specialty program through discharge. Such data will be analyzed on at least a semiannual basis for trend identification and incorporation into the ongoing continuous quality improvement program. Use this information to identify opportunities to improve services to the underserved of the community and to improve the outcomes of services provided to patients.

Policy

It is the policy of the hospital to maintain accurate records of referrals to the continuum services.

Procedure

Upon referral to the specialty program, the prospective patient's name, actual referral source, time and date of referral, physician, medical diagnosis, payor, and site will be entered on the log sheet (see Figure 9-1). The time and date of prescreen evaluation, if applicable, will be added to the form, as will the admission decision.

> **Guide to using the form:**
> 1. Patient name
> 2. Time and date of referral
> 3. Physician (patient's primary physician)
> 4. Medical diagnosis (primary, secondary)

Referral Date and Time	Patient Name	Referral Source	Physician	Diagnosis 1, 2	Payor	Site	Prescreen Date and Time	Admit Y or N

Figure 9–1

5. Payor

6. Site—where patient is to be evaluated (i.e., hospital and room number)

7. Actual referral source—individual responsible for referral (may be obtained during prescreen evaluation)

8. Time and date of prescreen evaluation

9. Admission decision—accept (Y), deny (N), reason

Policy

It is the program's policy to maintain accurate records of admissions and discharges into the continuum services.

Procedure

The patient's name, age, admission date, location, physician, medical diagnosis, and payor shall be recorded on the admit/discharge log sheet (Figure 9-2).

The date of discharge, length of stay, and discharge destination shall be recorded on the log sheet upon patient discharge.

Guide to using the form:

1. Patient name and age

2. Admission date

3. Location

4. Physician

5. Diagnosis

6. Payor

7. Discharge date

8. Length of stay

9. Disposition

HOW TO USE THIS INFORMATION

Maintaining logbooks for this information is only the beginning. Tabulate the information, review it at least once a year, and update it annually.

Patient Name and Age	Admission Date	Location	Physician	Diagnosis	Payor	Discharge Date	LOS	Disposition

Figure 9–2

PREPARING THE ANALYSIS

If you have developed a format very similar to the one we provided, you will want to aggregate the material as follows (as a minimum):

- Referrals by month
- Admissions by month
- Conversion rate per month (what percentage was actually admitted)
- Referrals by physicians (profile sheets, what diagnoses, etc.)
- Admission by physicians
- Conversion rate by physician
- Referral driver sources (physician, hospital based, family, physician office staff, etc.)
- Referral sources: location—(Hospital A, Hospital B, Clinic X, home and family, skilled nursing unit (SNU), nursing home, etc.)
- Tours conducted and by whom (conversion rate)
- Reasons for "did not admit"—denials

Also chart hospitalwide admissions by month to see the big-picture trends.

WHAT THIS INFORMATION CAN REVEAL

Area of Analysis: Potential Information and Opportunity

Referrals and admissions by month	Trends, planning campaigns, and blitzes during traditional periods of seasonality; these are also helpful in managing staffing.
Conversion rate by month	Types of referrals at various times of year, conversion rates should be compared across different periods of occupancy. If occupancy is 100 percent, where are the referrals being routed and do they receive appropriate care?
Referrals, admissions, and the	What types of patients do they refer? Are they appropriate? Do

conversion rates by physician	they need education in specific areas? What is the success of the marketing effort?
Referral sources: "drivers" of referrals (actual referral source)	Who is actually responsible for referrals? Is your pattern in keeping with national norms, your targets, and the maturity stage of your specialty program?
Reasons for "did not admit"	This is possibly more important than why patients are admitting. Are community needs unmet because certain program components or locations are missing? Do misconceptions exist and is fine-tuning thus indicated for the marketing plan?
Tour conversion rates	Identify those who can truly sell the program and, conversely, those who can most likely benefit from further education.

SAMPLE INFORMATION FROM A LOGBOOK REVIEW

We have included a few of the pages from a review of an acute rehabilitation hospital (Figures 9-3–9-6). There is not a complete year of information in this particular review, making trend analysis impossible. The most important issue to remember in performing analysis is the basic concept of the quality of information. The saying "garbage in, garbage out" is never so true as in analysis. In our review of inquiries, referrals, and admissions, our first suggestions are often about recordkeeping. This area encompasses both the actual recordkeeping and the maintenance of the documents. However, there is always something to be gained by even a partial review of the records. You may find assessing just what these records say to you interesting. An effective marketing plan for a specialty unit or program cannot be developed without an understanding and a constant review of the implications of referrals and admissions.

The focus facility is an acute rehabilitation hospital in the South. The facility had been open for some time but had not kept adequate records. The new admissions coordinator had begun the recordkeeping process. We were approached by the regional vice president of operations for the parent corporation and asked to review referral processes. The regional officials believed that given the competition, location, and other specifics of the market, the facility should have a higher census than it had. No inquiry information was recorded and we could not identify what if any issues in this area were causing a loss of referrals. The referral logbook gave us limited information because referrals were not kept by diagnosis and could only be pulled individually by every face sheet on patients who were admitted. We could not ascertain if any specific diagnoses were being lost. Figure 9-3 indicates the referrals by month for the months October through June.

Within nine months the facility had received 706 referrals. Although many rehab facilities see a decline in referrals in December (the traditional end-of-year holiday periods and summer months are often referred to as "seasonal census" periods of time of lower patient population pool), this facility had experienced a rise in referrals. A review of marketing plans indicated that the facility had been proactive in seasonal planning to alleviate census swings in November and December. The marketers had conducted blitzes to ensure that they received a greater market share during this time period to maintain census. January is traditionally a period of high census, as is February. Referrals to the facility fell in February. A review of census sheets

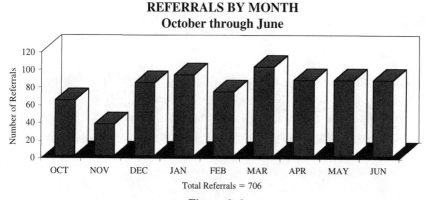

REFERRALS BY MONTH
October through June

Total Referrals = 706

Figure 9–3

indicated that the facility was at almost capacity occupancy in February (see Figure 9-4); marketers backed off promotion so that they would not create demand that could not be satisfied. Referrals remained steady through the month of June.

In reviewing admissions by month we were disappointed to see that only 67.9 percent of referrals were admitted (see Figure 9-5). This conversion rate is derived by dividing the number of admissions by the number of referrals. The goal for this facility was 80 percent; given the location and the fact that the facility was the only rehabilitation hospital in the area, this should have been achievable. Several issues were identified as we interviewed staff.

Many of the referrals were denied admission because they were at too high a functioning level to qualify for rehabilitation. The liaisons who screened patients asserted that hospital-based discharge planners were not proactive in referring. Other referrals did not convert to admissions because they were from rural families and decided just to go home. The number of admissions was suspiciously constant, hovering between 55 and 62, with the exception of one month. We would have expected more fluctuation with changes in patient population pool.

We made a number of recommendations. We will confine our discussion to only a few here.

- Market more aggressively to hospital-based influencers and referral sources to increase knowledge about acute rehabilitation.

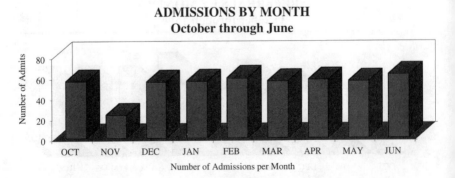

ADMISSIONS BY MONTH
October through June

Number of Admissions per Month

Total Admissions = 480

Figure 9–4

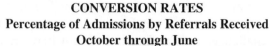

CONVERSION RATES
Percentage of Admissions by Referrals Received
October through June

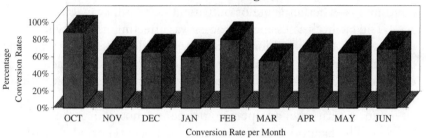

Average Monthly Conversion Rate = 67.9%

Figure 9–5

Use in-services and mailings of information on patients' progress to referral sources in order to educate them about the benefits of rehabilitation.

■ Involve the acute rehab therapists with the hospital-based therapists to build referral relationships by educating them on how quickly patients can be moved to rehab. Formal on-site visits and phone calls regarding patients admitted to secure clinical information was recommended.

■ Increase physician marketing. Physicians are intermediate referral sources, meaning they may not have appropriate patients today but will sooner or later. If physicians are supportive of acute rehabilitation, they will refer appropriate patients. The written referral in the chart "refer to XYZ rehab hospital" is more likely to convert to a referral than a referral from social services that may be directed to multiple providers. This facility had concentrated all of its marketing efforts on social workers and hospital-based discharge planners and had not built a physician referral base. This contributed to patients choosing to go home without postacute care when they could have benefited from rehabilitation services. The physicians had not been sufficiently educated and were unable to recommend the services to their patients.

■ Phone referred patients/families who chose to go home to see if they are making a safe, healthy transition and to educate them that they may be able to access services if they find that they do need help. Patients who have chosen to go home often realize that significant challenges are in store but do not know that services in the continuum—whether acute or outpatient—are still available.

The facility's assessment process was affecting its ability to admit patients in a timely fashion. Staff were confident that they were the only rehab provider in town and did not view the skilled facilities as competition. The skilled facilities viewed themselves as competition for every rehab candidate and were often quicker to assess patients on-site and return the acceptance notice to hospital-based referral sources. The facility's assessment team members reported a two-hour review of chart and patient interview that the competition was often conducting by phone or with a brief chart review. When the rehab assessor finally went in to interview and "sell" the patients, they had already been visited by someone else and had often developed a relationship that facilitated transfer.

■ Revamp the assessment process, establishing a minimum time frame that will be acceptable for the patient to visit the facility and be screened. Reeducate the assessment team that the prescreening assessment is only a tool for determining admission, not an initial history and physical on the patient. The assessments were taking too long, which was curtailing the liaisons' abilities to screen more patients, conduct better follow-up to referrals, and market to referral sources. (When I visit with individuals who assess patients I always ask, "How many assessments do you perform per week on the average?" and then later in the conversation, "About how long does it take to perform an assessment?" With simple arithmetic, I can estimate the number of hours per week they spend on assessments and then determine what they do with the remainder of the forty-hour week.)

This facility did not track referrals by "driver"—that is, they knew what hospital the referrals were coming from but could not tell me who was actually responsible for the referral. (Refer to the previous comments about conversion rates of referrals driven by hospital-based referral sources vs. those driven by physicians). The referrals were predominantly through hospitals (see Figure 9-6).

Our recommendations were as follows:

■ Begin to identify the referral driver. This can be accomplished by having the assessment team members check the chart to determine if the referral was the result of a physician writing "refer to XYZ rehab" or "begin discharge planning." In this way they could determine who was driving referrals. This would be helpful in recognizing the success of the marketing effort if a targeted physician finally wrote "refer to XYZ rehab." It would also help in identifying hospital-based referral sources who needed further education about whether to refer patients to rehab or to other settings.

■ Educate physicians on the referral of patients from home and the office. Many facilities receive referrals from physician offices and are asked to assess patients in the home. This was not occurring at the focus facility. We recommended development of a campaign to educate physician staffs on this potential. We recommended that this campaign also be used at such events as health fairs, and in advertising, so that the public would be aware of this other referral opportunity.

Numbers only tell part of the story, but they provide a starting point to identify areas of concern and to develop strategies to address them. We encourage you to determine if complete and accurate records are maintained, but more importantly, if they are being used.

CENSUS MANAGEMENT PLANS—THE NEXT STEP

Now that you have studied the information contained within the tools accessible to you right in your own facility, it's time to put them to work for you. Many facilities work from annual marketing plans

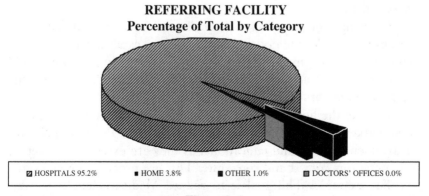

REFERRING FACILITY
Percentage of Total by Category

HOSPITALS 95.2%   ■ HOME 3.8%   ■ OTHER 1.0%   ▣ DOCTORS' OFFICES 0.0%

Figure 9–6

without assessing the admission trends of their hospital and local community and specialty units. This can lead to many problems including the following:

- Public promotion of programs just before or during traditional periods of high occupancy, which create staffing issues, demands that you cannot satisfy, and census for your competitors.
- Promotion of programs with associated expenditures at inappropriate times. An extreme example would be a focus on joint replacement during the period between Thanksgiving and end-of-year holidays.
- Missing the opportunity to build awareness at the exact time that there is increased potential for referrals to certain specialty programs. For example, during January and February, many rehab and skilled programs have increased orthopedic population.
- Attempting to schedule screenings with physicians during a period when they traditionally attend specialty conferences or take vacations.
- Failing to strategically select programs to be represented at health fairs when space at such events is limited.

The following are ways to make your plan a continuum plan:

- Develop and implement a different approach to planning, with quarterly plans and annual overviews from each specialty program (refer to Figure 9-7).
- Use the annual overview to develop the master calendar for the marketing department (refer to Figure 9-8).
- Be flexible and remember that the plans can change with market changes.
- Change the way your facility allocates marketing dollars. The allocation of marketing dollars should not be a catalyst for scheduling events and campaigns but rather a result of strategic planning. Build an awareness of strategy, rationale for resource expenditure, competitive positioning, and continuum contribution.
- Make the hospital's budget the marketing objective. The allocated marketing budget does not drive promotion. Promotional tools are as much internal and educational as they are external. Marketing and operations coexist and cooperate. This is a process, not an event.

For example: The goal is to reduce Medicare length of stay. Strategies will be to promote continuum of care services to employees

Specialty Program:

Year _____

Quarter:

☐ SNU   ☐ Cardiac rehab
☐ REHAB   ☐ Home health
☐ CORF   ☐ Adult day care
☐ Geropsych   ☐ Day treatment

☐ Jan - Feb - Mar
☐ Apr - May - Jun
☐ Jul - Aug - Sept
☐ Oct - Nov - Dec

QUARTERLY CENSUS-MANAGEMENT PLAN

Strategy Steps	Target Date	Person Responsible	Rationale	Actual Date

FIGURE 9–7

Specialty Program: Annual Overview

CENSUS MANAGEMENT EVENTS PLAN

	JAN	FEB	MAR	APR	MAY	JUN	JUL	AUG	SEPT	OCT	NOV	DEC
SNU												
Rehab												
CORF												
Geropsych												
Home health												
Adult day care												
Day treatment												
Cardiac rehab												

Figure 9–8

and physicians who will appropriately move patients into a more cost-effective level of quality care. Take the following steps:

- Prepare a hospital analysis of DRG runs to identify diagnoses of patients with longer-than-desirable lengths of stay and physicians who will be key to change. Identify discharge planning professionals assigned to floors or services to be involved.
- Instruct specialty program directors or marketers to target identified physicians with one-to-one educational efforts to change referral patterns and assess operational opportunities.
- Ensure that continuum unit staff are educated in providing quality care for those patients (with related diagnoses and service requirements) who will be targeted through the effort.
- Provide education opportunities and laminated cards to physicians on billing for specialty units.
- Educate unit staff in continuum services so that they may assist in efforts to families and physicians.
- Develop continuum brochures, order holders, and place them on the backs of patient room doors on appropriate units.
- Develop sticky notes for continuum referrals for the Utilization Review to use on patient charts.
- Restructure the discharge planning process to include developing routing systems through the continuum, not single referrals.
- Develop public education presentations or campaigns related to this continuum.

SUMMARY

We recommend first analyzing the internal situation and any necessary restructuring of the process to focus on the continuum of care and what it means to the facility or system, the patient, and the payor. Although many of us may have traditionally viewed marketing as separate from operations, in truth they are interdependent. The successful facility must destroy the "my program" wall that was built over the years and replace it with "our continuum."

10
CHAPTER

Strategic Placement of the Healthcare Client

Paula Lodes

As healthcare evolves into the year 2000 and beyond, the challenge facing the healthcare professional is to place their patients strategically within an evolving and ever-changing healthcare system. The task becomes to create that seemingly magical blend of physical, functional, and mental capabilities at the appropriate healthcare level at the right time and place. Occasionally, all these factors proceed without incident. The patient travels through the system and the outcome is a healthier patient, a satisfied family, and a nonstressed healthcare professional. Of course, we always begin the process with hopes for optimal outcomes for all parties.

More often than not, this doesn't happen. Assisting the patient through the appropriate pathway lends itself to many challenges for all involved. And challenges exist within the healthcare system itself. Services and pathways differ from one area to another and in fact from one hospital to another. The system has changed so drastically over the past decade that it has yet to catch up with itself.

So how do you strategically recommend a particular pathway that is advantageous to the facility as well as to the patient? How do you educate and motivate the team of healthcare professionals consistently to recommend pathways targeted to satisfied customers, address patient needs, and meet proposed budget goals? What factors determine what level of care is appropriate? What avenues exist for the patient to progress? Furthermore, how do you uniformly provide the patients and family with quality workable solutions to their growing needs? In this chapter, we will provide a method of searching for the answers and a glimpse into successful solutions to these multifaceted problems.

First and foremost, the healthcare system must provide patients with pathways through the system. These pathways must contain methods by which the patients and their families are kept continually educated regarding their options. Most healthcare agencies have elected to implement case-management services using registered nurses as key coordinators. These specially trained nurses use both clinical and administrative skills to coordinate pathways through the system.

Case management is not a new concept to healthcare. It has proven itself consistently in years past. The RN case manager should be selected with utmost care, since this position has the potential of making or breaking the system. A perfect fit, if chosen correctly, will prove valuable. Case managers should have exceptional clinical skills and should communicate in terms easily understood. They are also given the job of educating the patient and the family about the clinical situation and the perceivable outcomes. They must be knowledgeable of the various phases of the system. The case manager must possess a workable understanding of the criteria of each level of care as set forth by Medicare and other governing agencies. A successful case manager also borrows concepts from the fields of marketing and public relations to guide the patient and family strategically through this complicated system. Certainly, and most importantly, case managers must exhibit a gentle, positive nature. Please commit these points to memory as we later address the issue of educating healthcare professionals about particular pathways.

"One step at a time" is often used as a statement of wisdom. It also lends itself to a potential direction within the healthcare system. However, patients within the system are more commonly subjected to multiple steps taken in multiple directions and without explanation. This results in confused patients and family members, and a frustrated team of healthcare professionals. Steps can be taken to eliminate some, if not all, of the sense of frustration and confusion even though we cannot prevent or avoid all of it. Please consider the following array of interrelated models as a method of explaining this somewhat complicated process.

MODEL OF INVOLVEMENT CONCEPT

First, let us examine a simple concept, referred to in this text as the *model of involvement* (see Figure 10-1). It is a method of identifying all parties who communicate as the patient passes through the system. But what seems to be simple is often the most difficult to accomplish. At the close of several team conferences involving the patient, multiple family members, and a score of healthcare professionals, I have wondered who the patient was—the one supposedly being treated? Even though this might sound ridiculous, the fact remains that there can exist more than one patient in each scenario. But for identification's sake, the patient is the one wearing the "fashionable gown."

Model of Involvement

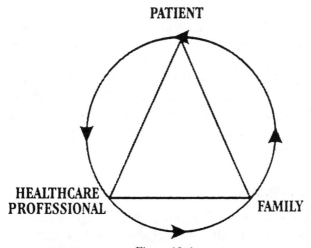

Figure 10–1

P. Lodes 1996 (illustrated by B. Buttry)

Family members or significant others must also be identified. The establishment of communication early after admission of the patient is vital in a successful transition.

The evolution of the family unit has proven challenging over the past decade. In years past, families cared for their aging, and in some cultures this is still important. However, the American family unit has evolved somewhat from this earlier picture. With the modernization of transportation and the versatility of American business, the once tight-knit family unit has stretched its boundaries beyond the horizons. This creates many problems. Siblings are miles apart and working seemingly endless hours, cannot relocate regardless of the situation. The parent (usually the patient), on the other hand, is not always willing to relocate closer to the children.

In these situations, patients are now having to implement alternative solutions to problems once addressed by the family unit. As you can imagine, the financial component now becomes an issue. Multiple phone conversations must be initiated by the case manager apprising the family members of each move within the system. The family members comprise the second point of the triangle within the circle of communication.

The third and final point of the triangle is the healthcare professional. Ultimately, the healthcare professional should be identified as a team of professionals. But often, realistically and somewhat unfortunately, this is only one person. The team approach, used most consistently in the rehabilitation phase of the healthcare system, is a preferred method of addressing complex problems, with a far wider scope. Research has substantiated that clear functional pictures are derived from the input of several varying sources. In lay terms, "two heads are better than one." The team should consist of the physician, dietary, therapists, nurses, and social services professionals. Together, the can construct and implement strategic, well-planned informed decisions from all aspects.

MODEL OF APPROACH

Informed decisions are implemented with care and accuracy. Perhaps arriving at the end of a well-constructed plan is the result of a strategic road map of options. The *model of approach* will help simplify the process by which informed decisions are constructed (see Figure 10-2).

Model of Approach

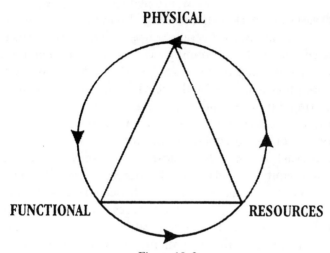

Figure 10–2

P. Lodes 1996 (illustrated by B. Buttry)

During the acute phase of hospitalization, the patient's physical condition remains the top priority. It must be stabilized. The term *acute* refers to the patient's initial admission into the healthcare system. As most of us are aware, revolutionary change has occurred in the acute phase of the system. Since the implementation of the DRG payment system by Medicare in the mid-1980s, the time spent in the acute phase of hospitalization has been decreasing. Currently, some areas of the United States are experiencing two- to four-day lengths of stay. This approach requires patients to be swiftly stabilized from their acute illness without unwelcome events. The team players most important at this level of care are the physicians, nurses, and the case manager. Careful attention must be paid to the patient to ensure rapid stabilization of the medical problems and to prevent recurrence. The acute length of stay, whether it is of the Medicare patient, insured patient, or the managed care participant, is becoming increasingly critical in the continuum of care pathway.

The second point of the triangle within a circle of communication is the patients' current level of function and their proposed needs based on that functional level. Again, the team approach is the most effective way to determine function. Therapists are instrumental in doing this, as well as in training patients and their families how to overcome obstacles. It is crucial at this point to stop and evaluate the patients' future potential. Illness, accidents, and disease processes can leave a devastating mark on the patient. What is a simple task to a normal functioning adult can become a frustrating, worthless act of uncoordinated function. Determining a course of events and implementing a secondary backup plan are well worth the time and effort spent. The disease process coupled with the patient's attitude and motivation often determine the best-laid plans.

Last, and perhaps most important, what resources does the patient have to put into effect? Resources can be from two varying sources: internal (functional, physical, motivational, etc.) and external (family, community, financial, etc.). Resources will vary from one community to the next. Case managers will become experts on the resources available to the patients in their area. In some instances where patients are being moved from one location to another, the case manager in conjunction with the patient and family will jointly make arrangements. But resources within communities are dwindling, especially to those whose financial status is poor. This reminds me of a case that involved moving a stroke patient from an acute care setting in a Nevada hospital to a rehabilitation center in the patient's home state of Oklahoma via military transport. After several days and many phone calls, the patient began her journey. It took two days with layovers in five states.

The model of involvement and the model of approach merge to create two intermeshed circles of communication. Alterations in any angle within the triangles of the intermeshed circles cause the result or outcome to be skewed, creating a less than perfect outcome. This could result in the patient being placed hastily at an incorrect level in the continuum and receiving less than adequate care. In other instances, skewing of the communication circles could result in dissatisfied customers of the healthcare system and render them apprehensive in future encounters.

To provide consistency, a look at the various pathways within the healthcare system is beneficial. After the patient has been transferred or discharged from the acute care setting, the patient and the healthcare team have several options based on the model of approach components. Most patients prefer to be discharged to their home, to return to their physician's office in a few days or weeks. This occurs in the best of situations. If the patient requires additional monitoring and is considered to be homebound, home health services are available to assist. Services provided in the home health arena are nursing services and physical, occupational, and speech therapy, as well as specialty nursing services including pharmacological interventions. The criteria for discharge of the patient from the home health service are outlined specifically by Medicare, insurers, and managed care providers. Outpatient services are an option for those patients who need continued care and who are at a level of functional independence. For involved cases requiring additional time for medical stabilization, the patient may be transferred from the acute setting to a skilled nursing bed. These are commonly referred to as skilled nursing units, skilled nursing facilities, and, in some instances, subacute services. These services are now offered by many sources ranging from hospitals to nursing homes. The patient must qualify for skilled nursing using criteria set forth by Medicare. If an acutely ill patient requires a longer period of time to recover, a long-term care facility may be the best solution. Family members should be actively involved in locating a long-term care facility that will adequately address the needs of their loved one and is within a convenient distance. Acute comprehensive rehabilitation programs (inpatient) are specialty programs focused on helping the patient return to a prior level of function. Neurological disorders are often addressed at this level of care. However, rehabilitative services are certainly not limited to this diagnosis. Inpatient rehabilitative care is available for patients whose functional potentials warrant fine-tuning. In most cases, functional outcomes are greatly enhanced with the implementation of a quality interdisciplinary rehabilitation team approach. This process can be carried through into the home environment with the implementation of home health services or in an outpatient setting referred to as a comprehensive outpatient rehabilitation facility (CORF).

Hospitals and healthcare agencies have joined with physicians to develop specific pathways for their patients to progress through the system. These pathways are complete with step-by-step interventions and specific predetermined time lines. This is in an effort to provide consistency throughout all aspects of the system. These highways of care are often referred to as *critical pathways* and are specific to each diagnosis. The future healthcare system will ultimately shape these pathways into lean machines as the healthcare dollar continues to shrink.

Having considered determining factors that plot the client's pathway, how then do you build a healthcare team of professionals who are synchronized with consistent quality care? One solution is to educate healthcare professional on a continuous basis. Because the healthcare system is continually changing, education of the professional must also stress creativity and flexibility. Implementing such programs as "DRG of the Week," case-management rounds, CQI programs, and educational in-services have proven successful in motivating healthcare professionals to synchronize options offered to clients. Creativity is an advantage when addressing methods to harmonize these professionals.

A top-notch case manager, as previously mentioned, is the key to the success of patients progressing through the system. In part, the success of case managers is the willingness on their part to be objective about their own position. They must be flexible in viewing all sides of the circle of communication. They must focus on patients and their physical, mental, and functional levels. They must value the concerns of the physician in the care of patients and the implementation of their practice. Case managers must discover resources for their patients that are appropriate and will provide quality care. The family's need for care, resources, and knowledge about how to care for their loved one are important issues determined by the manager. The case manager must also play an integral part in the healthcare team striving to return the client to prior levels of functioning. Last, but certainly not least, the case manager must seek the healthcare system's administrative goals for financial responsibility. All of these points are deserving of the case manager's time, energy, and efforts. Considerable time must be invested in shaping and educating the manager in the physical and financial concerns of all involved. Building a one-to-one relationship with these important coordinators of care could prove beneficial in establishing referral development trends.

The concept of total quality management, often referred to in healthcare as continuous quality management or CQI, can provide important insights for the manager. A characteristic of CQI is its continuous flow of information circling back to its origin. Case managers need to be in contact with their former clients to determine if the plans they helped construct were indeed progressive and appropriate. Did the pathway they implemented for their patients work for them and their families? Feedback from these sources could serve as a guide in the decision-making process for case managers and the institutions for which they are employed.

Strategically placing clients within current healthcare system pathways can be challenging. Because of the nature of the system itself coupled with the complexity of patients' needs and resources, patients, families, and healthcare professionals are often overwhelmed. Changes in the American healthcare system have been met with a more dramatic emphasis on outcomes. This perhaps has been the greatest change in the field of healthcare. Is it positive? The answer perhaps is more appropriately addressed in terms of how this change is faced. Will it be with open minds or closed spirits?

The following are seven case studies illustrating patients' movement through the continuum of care.

CASE STUDY 1

The patient is a 75-year-old male who recently suffered a stroke (CVA). The previously independently functioning patient lives with his 68-year-old wife of forty-five years. She has experienced many health problems over the past year but is currently functioning independently. They reside in a modest two-story Midwestern home with a maximum of four steps up to the first floor. The patient's wife limits her driving to local travel. They have two children. The son—the older of the two—resides out of state with a large young family. He is unable to participate in the care of his father. The daughter lives only blocks away from the family home. She is employed but is able to assist if necessary.

The patient's physical status is improving. The large CVA of three days prior has rendered the patient with dense right-side hemiplegia and hemiparesis. The patient is incontinent and is having difficulty swallowing. His overall functional level requires maximum assistance of two caregivers for transfers and activities of daily living.

To place this patient in the proper healthcare level, first identify the key players in the acute care setting: the patient, his family, and the key healthcare professionals. Contact with the key players ideally should be made within twenty-four hours after admission into the acute healthcare system. Frequent communication among all parties involved should be maintained on an ongoing basis. The patient's immediate physical condition should serve as the guide for his travel throughout the continuum of care. The functional level and the patient's resources serve as additional factors to be considered. In this case, the patient is three days poststroke with major physical deficits and is progressing at a slow, steady pace. At the close of the third day, a plan should be in place to move the patient to the next level of care. Bear in mind that the patient must remain medically stable. Very aggressive healthcare systems would move this patient to the rehabilitation phase early, progressing him to the acute inpatient rehab team. In some cases, especially if the acute inpatient rehab bed can accommodate a longer rehab stay, the involved stroke case could progress nicely in this scenario. However, most commonly the patient could benefit from additional time in a subacute or skilled environment. This allows the patient time to stabilize medically and still provides the patient the therapy intervention of nursing, physical, occupational, and speech.

Based on the patient's functional progress, he may soon be transferred to the acute inpatient rehab level following his stay in skilled nursing. The focus of rehab will be to return the patient to his maximal functional level. In this case, the patient and family both wished to return to their home environment. The average length of stay for this type of patient in the rehab setting is approximately two and a half to four weeks, again depending on the patient's progress, medical stability, family support, and response to the acute rehab team approach. Focus should be directed toward integrating the patient into his former environment. The patient's resources should be carefully evaluated. Caution was exercised not to overwhelm the spouse, who recently experienced health problems. Home health services would be beneficial if the patient's transportation access is limited. Outpatient services, especially a team approach often found in a CORF, would prove helpful in this situation. Communication throughout the healthcare pathway is essential for smooth sailing. Patient and family education is also a necessity. However, with today's increasing budgetary demands, these services often fall victim to cutbacks. Regardless of the pathway taken by the patient and his family, the healthcare professional should remain in contact with the patient to provide important feedback. Care should be exercised to prevent complications and further extension of the stroke.

CASE STUDY 2

The patient is a 70-year-old female who underwent an intensive bowel resection with colectomy three days ago. She is progressing well. Her IV has been discontinued and she is tolerating a liquid diet. Although the adjustment to her new colectomy has been frightening, she is participating in patient education and care of her stoma. She is ambulating in the hallway for more than 100 feet with only minimal assistance. She lives alone, having lost her spouse only a year ago. Her children live out of town; hospital visits have consisted of close friends from her church.

Based on the information given in this scenario, it is apparent that the patient is progressing without unwarranted events. The patient does, however, have several identified needs. She lives alone and for a few weeks following the surgery will be homebound. Her friends would probably assist her with minor errands. She has several identified educational concerns regarding the care of the stoma. After discharge from the acute care setting, she would benefit from home health services. Home health nurses could routinely check her for symptoms of developing problems and address them promptly to prevent further complications. The nurses could also assist the patient in the care of her newly placed stoma and with any medication and nutritional concerns. If she continues to progress without incident, her home health services would be discontinued and the necessary reports sent directly to her attending physician.

CASE STUDY 3

A 46-year-old female was involved in a serious auto accident in which she sustained multiple fractures. Because of the nature of the complex fractures, patient was left non-weight bearing on both lower extremities for six to eight weeks. She also suffered a deep facial laceration requiring multiple reconstructive surgeries. The patient was employed at the time of the accident and had insurance coverage. The patient's supportive family included a spouse and two children, one of whom was still living at home. The patient's home environment, however, presented several concerns. She and her spouse resided in a mobile home. A maximum of ten steps were required to enter the home, and door facings were too narrow to allow wheelchair mobility.

The patient stabilized within five days in the acute setting. Case managers from both the hospital and insurance companies agreed on skilled nursing services to allow the patient additional time to recover. Problems with discharge planning arose because of the availability of her home to accommodate her wheelchair status.

Following four days of skilled nursing services, the patient was transferred to an acute inpatient rehabilitation program. The purpose of this transition was to educate her regarding her non-weight-bearing status, home evaluation with modifications as recommended by trained therapists, and strengthening of her physical condition both to alleviate complications and to provide her with some sense of independence.

During the patient's stay in rehab, the therapists and family members were able to have a ramp built at home. Interior doorways were widened to permit the passage of her wheelchair. The patient was educated on strengthening exercises to build upper-extremity strength. She was also educated on proper transfer techniques and preventative measures to alleviate pressure sores and the problems associated with decreased function. Nursing services taught the patient to care for external fixation devices holding intricate bones steady for healing. After two weeks in the rehab environment, modifications were complete at home. The patient was released home for her remaining six weeks of non-weight-bearing status. She returned to the rehabilitation center at the close of eight weeks to receive intensive gait and transfer training. The readmission length of stay was five days. Five months later, she returned to the same rehab center and was walking with only cane assistance.

CASE STUDY 4

The patient is a 66-year-old female who experienced a right hemisphere CVA. Her deficits seemed minimal. The patient's left arm below the elbow and hand demonstrated weakness and numbness that improved over her course in the acute care setting. The patient's speech was intact and intelligible. The patient seemed to be progressing without incident. On the third acute hospital day, the patient was evaluated for potential placement into an acute inpatient rehabilitation program. The patient, however, refused the service. After several discussions with her physician and family members, the patient convinced the physician to discharge her to her home. The home environment consisted of an excellent family-support system and resources appropriate for proper monitoring after discharge. The patient and family members were given appropriate referral contacts. The patient was scheduled for a follow-up visit with her physician in two weeks.

Two days later, the case manager of the acute hospital setting from which the patient had been discharged received a frantic phone call from the patient's family. "Mom just walked off the porch of her home and fell 4 feet!" Luckily, the patient was not injured by the fall, but serious deficits resulting from her recent stroke quickly surfaced. The patient was admitted to the acute inpatient rehabilitation program for the evaluation of serious cognitive, abstract reasoning, and depth perception deficits. Thus, even though the patient seemed to be safe, in reality her condition posed different, dangerous issues.

The patient did progress without further incident in the rehabilitation environment after only a relatively short length of stay. Emphasis was placed on her being able to recognize potentially dangerous situations and on methods by which the patient and family members could compensate.

The patient was discharged to an outpatient rehabilitation team in the hospital's cost-based CORF. Family members were responsible for the transportation. They were also involved in important family education. The patient's function in her left arm and hand slowly returned to normal.

The patient remained accident free. The principal goal of the CORF environment was to apply the comprehensive interdisciplinary team approach to the patient in the outpatient setting. Because of the complexity of this patient's deficits, this type of patient is appropriately treated most comprehensively under this service.

CASE STUDY 5

The fifth case study demonstrates the plan of action involved in the care of a long-term care patient. The patient is an 84-year-old male who suffered a massive bilateral hemorrhagic stroke. The patient, with multiple functional deficits, was admitted to a hospital-based skilled nursing unit. He had left-sided hemiparesis and hemiplegia, as well as complex speech and language disorders consisting of both receptive and expressive aphasia. His swallowing disorder was discovered only after he was diagnosed with aspiration pneumonia.

The patient required maximum assistance in all levels of care and was incontinent for most bowel and bladder functions. His wife resided in a nursing home. The family member remaining to care for the patient was a caring and supportive daughter who was devastated by her father's illness.

The patient was able to participate only minimally with physical therapy, tolerating fifteen to twenty minutes of chair activities. Likewise, his participation in occupational and speech therapies was also minimal. Because of the nature of his swallowing disorder, the surgeon placed a permanent feeding tube (PEG tube) into the patient's abdomen to ensure proper nutritional status.

After the patient's pneumonia stabilized and the appropriate dosages of antibiotics had been administered, he was transferred to a long-term care facility. His functional and participatory levels were so minimal that he could not tolerate even low-level therapy. Yet his physical condition had stabilized. Counseling and emotional support were offered to the daughter.

Long-term care facilities, also known as nursing centers, do have a role in the treatment of patients. The trend of long-term care facilities to address more complex patient conditions has changed over the past decade from maintenance to restorative. Most facilities do offer physical, occupational, and speech therapies to their clients. Many offer a subacute setting and an array of continuum components.

CASE STUDY 6

A 52-year-old mother of four was diagnosed with malignant breast cancer. After the radical mastectomy, CT and bone scans evidenced progression of the disease into surrounding bone and tissue. Postoperative day two found this patient with significant drainage and pain because of tissue manipulation to remove suspected lymph nodes for involvement.

Late on day three the patient progressed to a level of medical stability and was released from the acute care setting to her home with home health services. Although the patient was receiving oral medication for pain management, the pain was not being adequately controlled. After careful consideration and assistance of the home health nursing team, the patient's IV was restarted with an infusion pump of intravenous pain medication administered on a timed basis. Physicians began to develop a plan of care to address the progressing malignancy. The patient was scheduled to undergo outpatient surgery for the insertion of a central line to administer both analgesics and future chemotherapy agents. Once the patient was home, these interventions were monitored by the home health nursing staff.

Both the patient and family members needed patient education in the care of the central line, as well as postsurgical care of the drains and incision site. The home setting was the appropriate site for the patient to recover. Chemotherapy agents were administered on an outpatient basis and then later in the home environment, closely monitored by the nursing staff and physicians. Physical therapy was ordered as a part of the home health care plan to prevent further complications and improve overall endurance levels. The home health nursing staff also implemented a program of emotional and psychological support, scheduling regular visits by other breast cancer survivors. Within three months, the patient was able to participate in outpatient chemotherapy and radiation therapy on an outpatient basis with transportation provided by her supportive family.

CASE STUDY 7

A 95-year-old female experienced a fall which caused a complex fracture of her right hip. Surgical intervention secured the hip in alignment and provided a future weight bearing status permitting of functional independence. The patient's medical history was complicated by vascular disease and mild congestive heart failure (CHF). The patient had lived independently and enjoyed church groups and gardening. Her supportive family consisted of two daughters and one son, all living relatively close and helpful in discharge planning.

The patient progressed through the acute care setting experiencing only minimal confusion as a result of post surgical anesthetics. On the fourth post operative day, the patient was referred to the skilled unit for further recovery, stabilization/monitoring of the physical condition, and therapies. After ten days in the skilled setting, she remained medically stable. On the ninth and tenth days she maintained participation in three hours of therapy daily. The patient's goal of returning to her home or to a foster home remained consistent through her hospitalization. Her required functioning for this level of care would be at a supervisory level seventy five percent of the time and minimal assistance of twenty five percent for the remaining hours. (Foster care has developed as another tier within the healthcare system. It is privately reimbursed and is available in some areas of high managed care involvement. The individual must be able to ambulate to and from meals independently or with an assistive device, and must be continent of bowel and bladder at night.)

The patient was screened for the acute rehabilitation unit and determined to be a candidate based on the patient's goals, current level of functioning, and potential for improvement. The patient participated in four hours of interdisciplinary therapy daily, with a care plan focused on attaining the desired functional level. Therapists performed a home evaluation at the adult foster care home, so that the family and patient could address issues affecting discharge. Within sixteen days the patient achieved the level required for foster care and she was discharged on the twenty-first postoperative day.

Extensive community re-entry services were ordered for the patient at three times per week for a period of three weeks in her foster home. The patient qualified for home care because of her need for close supervision of medical management, being homebound and unable to participate in frequent visits to an outpatient setting. Six months later the patient still successfully resides in the foster home and is participating in her regular church activities, transported by her family.

11

CHAPTER

Internal Marketing Opportunities to Strengthen the Continuum of Care

Teri Webster

No one would dispute that the scope of the healthcare market has changed dramatically over the last decade. All types of healthcare providers are faced with the need to be more effective in marketing their services to the community. With the advent of preventive health programs, comprehensive outpatient centers, full-service home health services, ambulatory day hospitals, outpatient surgery centers, and subacute skilled units, combined with managed care implications for allowed venues of service, providers are forced to fight harder for a diminished market share.

Marketing staffs often work to create an external image of the organization's service capabilities that goes beyond the comfort level of the operations staff. This issue applies equally to hospitals, nursing homes, and all other healthcare delivery sites.

In an increasingly competitive market, healthcare operations cannot afford to fail to provide excellent service to any sector of the community. One highly publicized failure can severely impede an organization's success in attracting referrals or admissions. With this in mind, the marketers and operations personnel must agree on the definition of their service capabilities.

However, a coordinated effort is not as simple as having the chief operating officer meet with the director of marketing to hash out a plan to work together. First, a marketing plan must be developed by the organization's executive team, and that plan must accurately reflect operations capabilities. Next, information must be disseminated throughout all levels of the workforce. Though workers may not have the full view of why undertaking new services is important, they must at least understand their role in implementing new services.

Even in smaller organizations, the adage about the right hand not knowing what the left hand is doing applies. Perhaps more than in any other industry, in healthcare it is vital to the consumer that all the workers be up-to-date on new programs and services. A loss of consumer confidence can come from a feeling that there is poor internal communication.

Few healthcare workers would describe themselves as underworked. But they can be perceived that in large part this way because of several factors: staffing patterns based on average acuity of care, poor systems for staffing replacements, and limited availability of well-trained staff in some areas of the country. Most staff healthcare positions are task oriented; the individual worker sees only those tasks for which he or she is directly responsible. Limited training attention is given to the bigger picture of the healthcare environment or organizational goals. Management's failure to understand the vital nature of employees' acceptance of new product lines can prove to be a critical error in the products' implementation and continued success.

This chapter will explore the processes that any organization can undertake to market new services internally.

REORIENTATION TO THE ORGANIZATION

When new services are offered within an organization, all staff need to be oriented to what types of service will be provided. Staff who understand the details of a new program can assist in promoting the program to the community. Often the healthcare facility is one of the largest employers in a small community, and the retention of that business is vital to economic health. Employees often forget that their livelihood comes from the business and that it is their responsibility to promote that business. In this day of employee rights and consumerism, employees often make harmful comments about their employer and do so in a manner that destroys the community's faith in the services provided. Healthcare workers are often eager to talk about their work and the status of affairs with their employer. What they forget is that loose talk can result in a breach of patient confidentiality and a loss in public confidence. Healthcare agencies that turn this phenomenon around are those that realize the power their employees have to either hurt the reputation of the organization or to build it up.

EXAMPLE: JUST A LITTLE CARD

One facility in a small town took this concept so seriously that the administrator had laminated business-card-size "capability cards" made up about his facility for each of his 250 employees and physicians. At a staff meeting he passed them out and asked that each participant read them carefully. The cards were part of a marketing plan to promote the facility's outpatient programs. Each card had the hospital name and logo with a list of all programs and services offered. On the back of the card was the facility's referral line phone number, its address, and directions from the main highway. He encouraged the employees to keep the card in their wallets and to give it away to someone when talking about where they worked. (What he did not tell the employees was that the hospital was losing money on inpatient services and that its survival would depend on building an effective outpatient referral base.)

The administrator also gave cards to the physicians at a medical staff meeting. He did explain the financial issues to the physicians and emphasized the importance of keeping the facility open for the local community. The administrator was careful to give only one card to each physician and employee. He asked them to give their card to someone in the community. He told each of them that he would replace their card if given away. He used this strategy so that the cards would actually be carried in a wallet instead of stacked on a desk. The total cost of the cards was less than $200.

The administrator's intention was to create an involvement and sense of ownership for each employee and physician. After three months, the administrator noticed an increase in referrals from the local physicians who had been referring to an independent outpatient clinic. He also noticed an increase in clinic use by his own employees and their families. The new business resulted in a 16 percent increase in the outpatient business in three months. Of course, the key was to retain market share and continue to increase it. But it is phenomenal to see an investment of $200 and employee and physician participation create new revenue of $7,200 in the first quarter. If the trend continued those cards would have produced $28,800 in new revenue in the first year, which was equal to almost two months of the facility's operating income before the cards were distributed. More importantly, if the facility provided consistently good service to the new clientele, the business would continue to grow from a good reputation in the community. The administrator took the card idea one step further and had the outpatient receptionist give one to new patients when they came to the clinic.

It should go without saying that all employees should be thoroughly oriented to the organization when they start to work. It is unfortunate that most organizations limit orientation to those issues that are regulated by the licensure boards (e.g., fire and safety rules and paperwork issues), and often fail to give new or part-time employees full tours of the facility. One marketing consultant who works with the long-term care industry advocates giving employees a tour and teaching each of them how to conduct the same tour. He believes that if the employee views it as his or her responsibility to be able to conduct a tour, then the visitor will never meet an unprepared staff member in the hallway when asking for directions.

The facility touring process should include and highlight only those areas that would be important to either the day-to-day work of the employee or to the visitor in making choices about which facility to use. Though many facility tour guides feel a need to show visitors the entire facility while spouting statistics, it is most important that the tour guide point out what applies specifically to the visitors' needs. Though no family member has ever refused to have their loved one admitted to a particular nursing home or hospital because the staff was too friendly and helpful, this issue also needs to be addressed during employee orientation.

Another consideration in reorientation of staff is making them aware of new or improved offerings. Refreshing the minds of staff members will help them remember what services are available. Recently a hospital lost its main therapist in the outpatient center. The therapist opened a competing outpatient clinic. When this happened the hospital briefly closed the center while searching for a replacement therapist. When the center reopened, referrals were going elsewhere and the center remained empty for almost a year. When it was determined that no therapist could be found and that the center was losing money and employees, the hospital administrator decided to use a contract agency to rebuild the practice. The administrator painted a dismal picture of the prospects of getting the business started again.

The first thing the contract agency did was hold a department head meeting in the center so everyone knew it was open. Agency representatives decided that the area needed to appear lively all the time by keeping the front curtains open, keeping the lights on, and having someone answer the phone on the first ring. Within weeks the center was getting referrals again. Next the agency staffed the center to accommodate a larger caseload so new referrals could pick the time they wanted to be seen. The receptionist began calling the local doctor's offices and reminding them of the center's office hours. Many of the physicians' offices responded that they had thought the center was closed. Within three months the center had more referrals than it could handle, and additional staff had to be added. This true story points out that a facility has to explore whether the community is transferring its loyalty to competing providers or whether it is simply failing to present qualified competition.

STAFF CROSS-TRAINING OPPORTUNITIES

Programs to cross-train line staff are rarely found in the healthcare industry. But while the cost of taking staff out of their regular positions and allowing them to learn what others in the organization do can be costly on the short term, it can reap some significant long-term benefits. Departments that are prone to complain about the contributions of other departments are often the best targets for cross-training. Not only will the cross-training likely reduce complaints, but it also will allow the staffs to get to know each other personally, thereby potentially further reducing complaints. Obviously, departments in a cross-training program must be complementary in the skill sets of the staffs for the training to be managed in a short time frame with any success.

A successful cross-training experience will achieve several objectives: (1) establish an understanding of the role of others in the organization, (2) promote an appreciation of the challenges of another position, (3) secure employee-developed ideas on improving interdepartmental procedures, and (4) build informal relationships that create a team perspective. Other potential advantages to cross-training are

(1) creation of a horizontal career ladder and (2) a more global perspective on organizational goals and coordinated efforts necessary to achieve those goals.

EXAMPLE: EVERYONE IS A LIAISON

One example of a successful cross-training experience can be found in an acute rehabilitation hospital (ARH). In an ARH, staff nurses are a vital part of the daily patient care team. Nurses also are used in a liaison role for community education and preadmission evaluation. The role of the liaison nurse requires a thorough understanding of the rehabilitation process, Medicare guidelines, and excellent skills in assessing patients. Liaisons are responsible for development of alliances with local referral sources that result in referrals to the ARH. Their responsibility also includes an assessment of patients (candidates) before admission to the ARH to determine their rehabilitation potential. The role of the staff nurse is to provide quality care to the patients once they are admitted. Though the basic educational requirements are the same for both positions, the experiential qualifications differ greatly. The staff nurse must possess the clinical skills to provide nursing care as a part of an interdisciplinary team. The liaisons must also have the clinical skills to assess patients but also possess the ability to educate the patients on the merits of choosing this particular ARH.

In this ARH, as is typical in hospitals, the reporting structure for liaisons and staff nurses had no common functions. The liaison department, comprised of clinicians, reported to their department head, who was responsible for marketing and case management. The department head reported to the vice president for marketing. The nursing staff reported to unit supervisors and then to the director of nursing.

The conflict between the two departments arose on several issues. First was the belief of the staff nurses that the liaison staff was compensated at a higher rate for a more cushy job. This belief resulted in part because the liaisons wore suits and carried briefcases rather than wearing scrubs and carrying clipboards. Second, the liaisons often supported the admission of patients who were difficult for the staff nurses—for example, patients with behavior problems or patients who had physical attributes that required additional care (such as a patient with both knees replaced who weighed more than 450 pounds). Also creating conflict was the nursing staff's belief that the liaisons did not provide enough clinical information in written assessment notes to allow staff nurses to have a perfect picture of the patient's needs upon admission (such as the size and type of tracheal tube needed). Further complicating the conflict, the liaisons did not work weekends or holidays.

From the liaisons' perspective, the nurses were paid on an hourly basis and were only required to work an eight-hour day, whereas the liaisons were salaried and sometimes their days lasted ten hours or more. The liaisons also viewed the floor nurses as less skilled than themselves. This perception resulted from the recruitment practices of the department head, who insisted that the liaisons must have a minimum of five years nursing experience. During a nursing shortage, the director of nursing was forced to hire new graduates to work on the patient-care units.

The conflict between the departments was not readily noticed because the two departments rarely interacted directly. What was apparent and puzzling to the director of the liaison department was that whenever there was an open liaison position, none of the staff nurses applied. At a department head meeting the two directors talked about this. The director of nursing said that the frustrations of the nursing staff were about the performance of the liaisons. They agreed that each department had some valid concerns but that it was in the best interest of patient care to find a resolution that would allow the departments to work together with more cohesion. They agreed upon a two-tier approach to the problem: (1) All new liaisons who did not come from the facility nursing staff would undergo a rigorous orientation schedule that included multishift orientation in the nursing department. (2) Selected members of the nursing staff would be trained to perform the patient prevaluation process and would accompany a liaison nurse for three days.

The first step was to establish a nursing orientation for the liaisons so that they could become familiar with the operating processes of the staff nurses. Because all the liaisons maintained active nursing licenses, this process was expedited. The department heads agreed that each of the liaisons would work on the floor as staff nurses for three shifts over the course of the month and that these shifts would be during days and evenings. During this time, the liaisons would wear scrubs and would perform all nursing tasks except IV medication administration. Secondly, the department heads agreed to have each staff nurse in the facility work closely with a liaison for three days after completion of a formal four-hour orientation program with the director.

The two directors convinced the senior administrative staff that this plan would benefit the entire organization in that a backup staff would be available for either department. It was also believed that this process would result in better communication by each department and result in better patient selection and readmission nursing preparation for patient care.

To give every member of the staff an opportunity to participate, the department heads scheduled the liaison orientation during a time when the census was highest and no admissions were being accepted. A waiting list was in place and the liaisons rotated through their nursing orientation at a time when they could be most helpful to the staff nurses. During high census, the liaisons also were exposed to a time of the highest frustration among the nursing staff about issues that the nurses perceived as being caused by the liaisons.

Immediately the liaisons noticed the issues that the nurses had been complaining about. Patients with special needs were admitted but their preadmission screening forms said nothing about special equipment that would be required. In the case of a man with a special urinary problem, the equipment to change his catheter was not on hand. Though the central supply department put a rush order on the equipment and had it the next day, the problem could have been avoided if the liaison had written down his equipment needs before admission. It was also a good refresher for the liaisons to have to stand on their feet for eight hours a day and to have to run every time the call bell went off. Many of them had forgotten the stress level of being a staff nurse. Another revelation was that the staff nurses had to complete patient care and be available for about ninety minutes of team meetings daily, so they had to be organized to get all of their required tasks completed during a shortened workday. The liaisons seemed to empathize with this issue because it was a concern common in their own jobs.

The nursing staff also got a new perspective on the role of the liaisons. With hospitals pushing for shorter DRGs, a greater share of the candidates for admission to the rehab hospital were coming from other sites. Not only did the liaisons go to the local hospital to preevaluate patients, but they also went into nursing homes and patients' homes to visit. Some of the homes were in dangerous inner-city neighborhoods. This was just part of the job for the liaisons, but it made a number of the staff nurses uncomfortable. Each of the liaisons was responsible for development of a referral base within a target area. This meant that some of them traveled two to three hours one way to evaluate a single candidate. The nurses learned quickly that running an office out of their cars was not nearly as glamorous as it had at first appeared. Lunch at the drive through three days in a row, trying to drive while on the car phone, and getting lost en route to a new referral facility were all parts of the liaison job. The nurses also picked up quickly on the fact that the hospital chart often did not give the liaison all the technical equipment needs information.

In working together, these groups made some changes to the patient-assessment form used for readmission evaluation, adding a space for patient height and weight and including a special equipment section. A number of other useful suggestions came from the experience, but perhaps the most startling outcome was the recruitment potential for the liaison department. Within six months of the cross-training, the liaison department had hired three nurses from the facility nursing staff. These were the first three candidates from the facility staff since the liaison department opened four years before. Each of the new liaisons brought hands-on rehab nursing experience to the job, thereby increasing the validity of the preassessment information. The outcome was a better liaison staff and fewer interdepartmental complaints. All this resulted in improved patient care. What the staff realized was that no matter where they worked in the organization, everyone is a liaison and has a responsibility to improve patient care.

CREATING A WORK-GROUP ATMOSPHERE

Healthcare is perhaps one of the most specialized of professional fields. Each function of caregiving has its own professional affiliation. Managers in healthcare often only manage their own professional group. Therefore a manager may not have enough knowledge of how the professionals can work together to achieve the organization's goals of being financially profitable and providing quality patient care. Many health professionals do not understand fully the capabilities of the other team members. This phenomenon is particularly apparent in the relationship between occupational therapy and nursing.

It is well known within any healthcare setting that the nurse is the primary caregiver and the responsible party for the coordination of all patient services. Occupational therapy (OT) is less understood by most health professionals, due in part to its misleading name. OT focuses on the functional performance of the individual and their ability to provide self-care in the aspects of activities of daily living (grooming, bathing, dressing, and toilet use), feeding, and homemaking/maintenance skills. For the functional adult, these areas make up the capabilities that enable us to perform our daily duties. OT is a complementary profession to nursing but is perhaps least understood by nursing because it infringes upon the tasks with which nursing has long been associated. The crucial difference between OT and nursing is the approach. Nursing is facilitative in nature—to help patients put on their socks or to give them a bath, for example. OT focuses on adapting the method patients themselves use to put on their socks. OT breaks down the tasks involved in giving a bath so that the patient can do the task without assistance. The basic philosophy of these disciplines are different.

In the nursing home industry, Omnibus Budget Reconciliation Act (OBRA) regulations guide the nature of patient caregiving. Among the regulations is the expectation that a resident will not regress in functional capability. This regulation is fraught with challenges, beginning with the fact that most nursing home residents are elderly and will of course continue to age during their stay in the facility. Medicare provides an opportunity for residents to participate in occupational therapy. To further complicate matters, within the nursing home industry nursing is considered a part of the routine cost limit (RCL) that sets the daily reimbursement for room-and-board services, but occupational therapy is exempt from the limit. It can be provided as an add-on service with Medicare reimbursement. To most nurses it is difficult to understand why staffing levels have to be so low in the nursing department when there can be extra OTs whom Medicare will cover. Some may tend to feel that it would be better and more efficient for patient care to have more nurses who will get the job of bathing and dressing done with clockwork efficiency rather than having OTs who spend long hours trying to get the patient to do it. This conflict in approach can often set the tone for all nursing and OT interactions in the nursing home.

It takes an articulate and approachable OT to overcome these issues in most nursing homes. It also takes a willingness on the part of nurses to talk with the OT to determine together what can be done realistically to prevent a resident from deteriorating over time. The reality is that with the proper use of OT, the nursing caseload can be reduced. There is a difference, however, between getting the nursing department to accept OT and having the nursing department expect OT to bathe and dress all residents regardless of their ability to recover and retain function.

This is the type of intraprofessional challenge that faces the healthcare industry as a whole. It is incumbent upon healthcare administrators and operations directors to educate on how other disciplines can be tapped to help achieve a common goal for patient care. There is no easy answer to this issue because of its global nature. The challenge is to the multidisciplinary manager to understand and teach how all healthcare disciplines can complement one another.

CONCLUSION

From the smallest agency to the largest multifacility organization, it is vital that a corporate culture be created that invites all employees to work together. Whether the issue is coordination of patient care or marketing of the organization, the approaches are similar. First, by recognizing that the employees are the first-line community to be approached with any marketing effort, you assure continuity of the message to the larger community. Second, the organization must promote an inclusive philosophy that involves all employees by recognizing that everyone has a vital interest in the organization's survival. Third, the managers must work together to ensure that all departments are getting the global message that the individuals of the organization must achieve a cohesive approach to patient care. And finally, it must be understood that the goal of any healthcare concern must remain what is best for the patient's care. These are perhaps the hardest lessons any professional can learn because they must be lived and practiced rather than quoted from a book. Certainly there are more changes on the horizon for healthcare, and with them will come more challenges. The organization that is in touch with its community through its employees will be best prepared to face the future.

THREE

EXTERNAL STRATEGIES FOR THE CONTINUUM OF CARE

In chapters 12 through 21 our focus shifts from internal marketing of the continuum of care components to the external issues of marketing. First, we address techniques for marketing to the public and working with the media to promote the continuum. We can educate healthcare professionals to initiate referrals, but the public must have an existing knowledge of the provider that will validate the referral and convert it to an admission.

We include chapters on marketing to physicians, territory development, managed care, and competitive and process assessments, applicable to all continuum component marketers. Physician-driven referrals generally result in a higher conversion rate to admissions. Therefore the ability to effectively promote to physicians is paramount to the success of programs. Managed care also drives admissions because of the direction of patients to network providers. A knowledge of managed care is imperative not only to marketing to the payor but to working with physicians who are network providers. If our own internal systems are structurally sound and complemented by the marketing effort, we must then scrutinize the competition to be truly prepared in the marketplace. Chapters are added on assisted living and skilled care for those who may be facing this challenge. The final two chapters present samples of tools that can be tailored to different components and to assist the marketing manager in coordinating the effort across the continuum.

12
CHAPTER

Marketing Your Services to the Public: Find a Way or Make a Way

Jackie Anderson

WHERE TO START

What would a teacher know about marketing and public relations? Or a fitness instructor? Or for that matter, a degreed marketer eager to make a mark in the healthcare profession. You look at your target area and it's pretty large. You realize your budget isn't. You may have any of a number of titles: community relations coordinator, director of women's health, wellness coordinator, director of health resources—the list goes on. In my time in healthcare marketing, I've been tagged with all of the above and more. Titles are not very meaningful. There is always the bottom line. That is where the rubber meets the road.

Find or make a way to increase the census for your organization. Whether it is a physician's office practice, a hospital, a home health agency, a nursing home, or another organization, you have the mandate. Start with a plan. So, how much time should you spend on planning? In my experience, planning time is a luxury to fit in as you can. You need your primary set of tools and a flexible system. I've found that organizing my "car office" is critical. That means not only restocking my car but ordering my materials with adequate lead time. If I can offer one significant buzzword for this field of marketing, it would be *lead time*. More on that as we proceed.

DEVELOPING A SYSTEM

And your system? I continually refine mine. Because I am out making calls daily in metropolitan areas (and previously in rural areas), I keep logs on each contact in my portable accordion soft briefcase (about $8 at a local store). You may be fortunate enough to have your own laptop. Each geographic area has a manila folder for contact logs. Other file cases may contain stationery, forms, handouts, and related articles. Because I often give lunch in-services, I keep two twenty-four-inch square plastic organizers for paper goods, always stocked. And of course a few giveaway items are also very handy. Self-adhesive note pads and pens are still top requests. In marketing to the public, a particularly crucial area is the task of building physician contacts. Obtain a medical directory for your area and start researching potential new clients. Block out a geographical section and begin your call process. Some days it's hard to spot the patients in a medical office because of the steady flow of marketers. It seems that everyone has something to present to your contact. Of course, you hope that you can be convincing in the few minutes that you claim. So, what will make you different or better? I learned that I cannot simply sell my product. I have to offer my contact a benefit. One that has worked very well for me in marketing to the public is to offer free physician clinics at my facility.

If you can persuade your facility to allow a clinic and to help with initial advertising, you can do the legwork to make it happen. If you have a membership newsletter, you have an advertising tool. If you do not, simple printed flyers that are distributed everywhere can be very effective. We recently marketed a two-hour program with continuing education units, primarily by flyers, that yielded an attendance of 130 nurses and social workers. A mail merge of all your contacts will spread the word. Use any and all of these techniques, including an insert in the newsletter of your chamber of commerce. The charge is usually minimal. An advertisement in your local newspaper is a lot more costly but obviously reaches a much larger readership.

For example, we held a one-day free clinic for people with joint pain for an orthopedic physicians' group. Two physicians who competed for the same business joined forces. We filled a complete day of appointments, with each physician seeing more than twenty people. Organizing the event required several meetings with representatives of key departments including radiology, the medical director, and dietary. We needed eight volunteers to fill half-day time slots, with two of us attending all day. Luckily we had top notch volunteers from our volunteer auxiliary. Of the more than forty attendees that day, several became new patients for the two physicians and eventually became candidates for our physical rehab center.

Another avenue in marketing to the public relates directly to a physician base. Find a niche for one particular physician that greatly benefits the physician, the community, and ultimately you and your facility or organization. There are speaking programs already created for you. One example is a package from the American Academy of Orthopedic Surgeons. For the nominal cost of reprinting their slides, you have a show to take on the road. The printed copy includes handout and speaking material. We incorporated a ten-minute demonstration of chair exercises with some stretch and relaxation techniques. If that's not your forte, someone in your organization could probably assist with another program feature.

Your job is setting up the speaking engagement, handling the publicity, and following up on all details. Check the lightbulb on the slide projector, the layout of the room, and the sound system hookup. I always make one trip to the room where our physician or guest speaker will be presenting. This has varied from sessions at a school auditorium on a Saturday, where we had 130 attendees, to a choir room with only twenty participants. One such presentation, in a church gym with more than 250 people attending, was an especially productive event that also resulted in name recognition for our facility.

Another idea for community awareness is presenting monthly forums highlighting medical staff, interspersed with lay speakers. This can be very effective. And if you offer finger food at these forums you will fill your room to capacity. We had to start taking reservations. We held some of the forums in the early evening, with most starting around noon. Before we began the forums, I surveyed a few community groups with two sets of topics. The respondents ranked contents numerically. One set was medical, the other was psychosocial. The local business women's club, my exercise class, and a board for a health foundation of which I was a member were my focus groups. The local chamber of commerce and organizations or clubs where you have some affiliation will usually allow a few minutes for a survey. Short and simple—the respondent applies number ratings to the items and it's done. That's the key.

Medical topics included laparoscopy (fairly new at the time), plastic surgery, cancer in women, and several other areas in which people wanted more information. Some psychosocial hits involved holiday food tasting and handouts on simple, easily prepared dishes. Another program topic was on laughter. The "laughter" speaker blew bubbles at the crowd in one segment of her presentation. You might say, "Great! So where do I find speakers? I can't pay the big bucks." In most cases the speakers I have invited speak for free or for under $100. You simply call everyone possible and determine who is already making such presentations. If your program is a free public service, speakers are inclined to reduce or eliminate their usual fees.

Once or twice a year, select a more well-known speaker. We had two fantastic speakers who were more than worth the extra expense. One spoke on the subject of first impressions. Another popular topic by a well-known local speaker was on personality analysis, featuring self-assessment handouts. Regretfully, we had to turn away several registrants. I'll never forget a forum on wok cooking where we took ninety-one registrations. Somehow we had overbooked, and at start time I saw about a dozen stressed people from a local club standing in the hallway. They could not be accommodated because we had failed to record all registrations. We scurried and borrowed chairs and squeezed them in, praying that we wouldn't have a fire-safety inspection that day. One extremely vocal gentleman, determined that his group would be seated, soon became one of our most faithful volunteers.

And that brings me to another important strategy for your consideration. Even if your organization does not have a volunteer auxiliary, you can still obtain voluntary workers. And if you do want to start a small auxiliary, you can get help. Volunteers are a very important resource. Anyone who discounts the services offered by older generations fails to realize their potential value. When I left one position in a hospital, a friend took over a membership program and staffed volunteers to assist. We met at one of our presentations and the next thing I knew, she was my right-arm volunteer. It is difficult to find paid workers who are as dedicated and dependable as some of the many special volunteers with whom I have served and had the honor to know.

Back to finding your niche in marketing to the public. Here is an example of a three-for-one win scenario. You can promote physicians, give your facility community awareness, and extend a service to your community. Establish a support group. Pick one that doesn't have a group meeting already established in your area. I have either started or facilitated about eight support groups. One that stands out is an arthritis support group. At one meeting, we staged a mock-up of a total knee replacement surgery. We had all the medical equipment, a gurney, each piece of hardware, the surgeon, a medical technician, another assistant, and a video camera displaying the surgery on a video screen mounted where the entire audience could watch. When the saw started cutting, you could almost feel the electricity in the air. Evaluations from our thirty-eight attendees were outstanding. I'll never forget that experience and certainly they won't either. Our physician expertly discussed the procedure and alleviated the anxiety of many who would be facing similar surgery.

Frequently, people suffer needlessly because fear causes postponement of helpful medical procedures. They need information, and by using various aspects of their sensory awareness, we enable them to make beneficial choices. The knee-replacement demonstration was a success for the audience, the physician, the hospital, and the marketer. Can you do this overnight? Obviously not. But long-range strategies allow you to plan ahead while you carry on today's business. I always stay three months ahead on every presentation. In the past, I've usually had a year's worth of topics and likely speaking candidates, securing them for any upcoming engagements whenever possible. Occasionally, I've locked in a year's calendar for a particular setting, such as a support group. You will find that you undoubtedly end up with cancellations, so you need to have a plan B arranged.

BEING YOUR OWN MARKETING TOOL

That leads me to another marketing tool. *You* will be the speaker. "What? I couldn't do that," you might say. Simply make "yes I can" one of your frequent affirmations. Join the local Toastmasters Club immediately if you have doubts about speaking. Try topics in areas that you find interesting and about which you have a comfortable level of knowledge, and offer yourself as a speaker. You might say, "But, it's November and everyone set their calendars last summer." Great! Offer to be a substitute speaker when there is a last-minute cancellation. I've often made presentations with one day's notice because I have several topics that fit in with most civic, social, and senior organizations. Also, this is your opportunity to get the contact person's phone number so that you can call to get on next year's calendar. I have spoken to groups ranging in size from fifteen to more than 200 members. Amazingly, after a little practice, it's really no different from one to another.

I recall when I was an at-home mom and I decided I wanted to become a fitness instructor. After months of perseverance, I made the grade and was hired to be a substitute exercise instructor. My challenge: How do you exercise, speak through a handheld microphone and try to captivate your audience so they will come back again and not drop out? I had never spoken before an audience in my life, unless you count school plays. So every day I turned on the television, cut the sound, and spoke to the TV people, as if they were my audience, working out the entire time. The day finally arrived. At the time, I lived in St. Louis and there was a blanket of snow over ice. It was too late to cancel exercise classes and one regular instructor could not make it. The voice on the other end of the line pleaded, "Will you please come?" My vehicle and I slid to the class, my heart in my throat. I think I secretly hoped no one would show, but they did! Three moms, four kids, and no nursery keeper. We did it, laughed, worked out, and were exhilarated! That was all it took. Take a few risks. Your self-confidence will soar! Courage comes with tiny starts. "I'm new at this job and I don't even know what community clubs there are in this area," you say. Your local chamber of commerce is a great resource. Visit and get to know the staff. They have booklets that you can have for the asking, or for a small fee, that list all the businesses, clubs, and organizations with addresses, contact people, and phone numbers.

Chambers of commerce, Lions Clubs, Rotary Clubs, Business and Professional Women's clubs, country club organizations, church senior groups, AARP, school PTAs, and local social clubs are among the organizations for whom I have presented. I do not have a long list of credentials. I am an unknown but I can offer a free benefit. It does not happen overnight. You meet people, you win trust and respect, and you work for an excellent organization. That's all you need to get in the door as a presenter. You tell your contact person up front, "I will be glad to speak on (the topic) and I would like three to five minutes at the meeting's end to give these handouts and mention my organization." You always get the agreement up front.

Right now you find yourself saying, "All right, fine. I can do this. But I'd like to do something unique, something that no one else is doing."

During my early days in healthcare marketing, a friend mentioned that she had heard about a great health spa. You could have a getaway weekend with one overnight at a reasonable price and enjoy herbal baths, massage, wraps, and a litany of other luxurious events. I went, I experienced, and I was conquered. So, how could I offer this to our community, give our hospital great press, and not have it dent my budget?

After a little negotiating with the spa management, we put together a weekend package. We did use the newspaper this time. By the target date we had forty registered attendees who met at our hospital Women's Pavilion at 9 A.M. on a Saturday. We served coffee and pastries, then checked our list. The group, one other marketer and myself, drove to the spa, which was only about twenty-five minutes away. Each person, including one married couple, checked in for their spa weekend. Meanwhile, we delivered a fresh rose in a vase with a handwritten welcome note to each person's bedside table. Everyone had a schedule of events, with optional leisure time throughout the two-day visit. Special services, such as massages, had fees that everyone knew about up-front.

We mailed complete information packets to each inquirer early in the advertising time line. We were able to offer exercise classes, relaxation classes, and stress management classes as free extras because my co-worker and I taught those routinely as part of the hospital wellness program. But you can find friends and associates who will help you in these areas. They just need lead time. The event was a great success, with many thank-you letters from our guests. The CEO of our hospital then asked me to repeat it for nurse managers as a thank-you for their dedication to our hospital. (It helps to have a progressive administrator.) Maybe a spa weekend is not something you want to do or is not possible because of demographics. However, your community offers many types of opportunities waiting for your creative ability. One of the best events we offered in our senior membership program was a day outing on a large paddleboat at an area lake. You always bring your guests to your facility and offer a small repast before you embark.

If you are marketing for a hospital, do you have a medical office manager's organization? If not, meet with your physician relations person and see if there is any interest in this type of program. Be involved and initiate a tour of your facility, particularly in any of your specialty areas. It is surprising how many physician office staff members do not know what your type of organization has to offer. And of course everyone will discover that seeing is believing.

EXPANDING YOUR TERRITORY

Suppose you want to crack open a new territory. For a variety of reasons, perhaps potential referrers and patients do not see you as a viable choice. I called on physicians and hospital staff in one such area when I was marketing a physical rehabilitation unit in a hospital. It was a forty-five-minute drive, and I could see eyes glaze over when I touted the benefits of our center. Yet I kept asking questions and listening, and then the idea finally snapped into place. Find a way, or make a way to transport patient families for visitation to see a patient who's in for a typical three-week stay. After many phone calls, appointments, closed doors, and sheer digging, the package was finally complete. We formed an arrangement with a county agency for vans and drivers and the transportation element was in place. Now I had the tool I needed. It started with one referral. It always does. Before long, there was a steady stream of referrals from that community. Word spread. Physicians talked to physicians. Better yet, patients and families told their friends. We had a small unit, but we stole business from many of our bigger competitors. Why? Because we offered a new solution to an old problem, and partly because the entire time that I was out marketing we had quality people inside our rehab unit giving personalized customer service.

    Our program manager was an innovator and a doer. When I asked, "What about white tablecloths on the dining tables?" it happened. Never mind that we set up our evening meals in our gym. Because of a full house, we could not accommodate everyone in our regular dining area. The unit had never had a full census before, so it had never been a problem. When our guests told us they felt as if they were in a hotel, those white tablecloths more than paid for themselves! Great marketing has to be a team effort. And again, it doesn't happen overnight. If your staff perceives you as a team player, helping wherever possible, whenever asked, you will find a reciprocal benefit. That is, then when you ask for help, you also get it. It all starts with giving first. We were a well-oiled machine. And even when the hospital census dropped, the rehab unit stayed full. Morale and motivation flourished.

And speaking of a team, try this. Pick a holiday and volunteer your services for that day. Eat with the patients and families, do the little extras: get a newspaper for a patient, run an errand for another person, chat with patients who are all alone that day, be a good listener if a patient wants to reminisce. It will be one of the best days you will ever have. Is that really marketing? You bet it is! It will not feel like it, look like it, sound like it, or taste like it, but it definitely is.

What if you look around and you say, "OK, I know how to market, but our competitors have many features that we don't offer. They have a luxurious setting and we're on such a tight budget." At our rehab unit we were constantly hearing the objection, "But you don't have water therapy." When I left the facility, we were in the midst of setting up a contract at a nearby therapy outpatient center with a pool. *Find a way or make a way.* At another new facility, we had bare walls inside the center. I pleaded for decorator art and pictures, but the controller said, "Right now, we do not have $3,000 for this enhancement." I bargained for $350 and went to a local mart and negotiated a deal on preframed, inexpensive prints. I brought them to the facility and let our team decide where to hang each picture. The *team concept* is so vitally important. Next, I went to the volunteer board and negotiated for an aquarium with one year of maintenance. I had all the information, with quotes from local vendors, when I presented the idea to our board. Usually, you just have to ask. And sometimes ask again. And again. But as marketers, we know determination. We must be proud of what we market and show ownership.

Every time you get a no, cheer. Because you're that much closer to a yes. It could take being told no nine times to get a yes. I loved no. I counted on it. How could I get to a yes faster? Call on more people and get those no's under my belt. Never take a no personally. Just cheer. I am that much closer because yes is just around the corner.

"Fine! Great! All these events and programs sound terrific. But I have no advertising dollars," you say. No problem. Can you afford colored paper and do you have someone in your organization who knows how to use a word processing graphics program? Now you have flyers to distribute everywhere. Since your events are almost always free to the public, learn to use resources such as local libraries, pharmacies, your facility lobby and waiting areas, physician offices, social service contacts, social and civic organizations, bulletin boards at grocery stores, church bulletin boards, and church bulletins. You just need good lead time. Always have a time line and take the time to plan ahead.

You say, "But my competitors do newspaper advertising. I can't afford it." Can you afford free? At one facility I counted thirteen target communities apart from our city that I wanted to market. I visited the editor of every newspaper in each town. Of course, that's not difficult with towns of 5,000 to 15,000 people, but I also managed to do the same networking in two towns of 60,000. I explained that I would be hosting events and presentations that involved their local populace. I told editors that I would periodically be sending black-and-white photos and short copy to them for any such event. That could mean that one or more people in their town attended some event at our hospital or it could mean an event held in their town.

I always had black-and-white film and a camera ready. Some editors wanted an undeveloped roll, others wanted negatives, and a few just needed the prints. You won't get them back unless you are able to make special arrangements and return promptly to pick them up. I was usually satisfied with reprints of my photo or article. Or I used two rolls of film. The first set went to the newspaper, and I would either send a second roll back to the audience or save it for the hospital scrapbook. This would be a colored roll. In my two-and-a-half years of marketing at that hospital, every article that I submitted went to print. You've practically become a free freelance reporter for the newspapers. We never paid one dollar for those publications. They were there for the asking. And after a while, our volunteers trained themselves to bring me the newspaper photos or articles, and I didn't have to drive back to each of the towns. Editors are usually much too busy to send you a copy, so I have always tried to be user-friendly and not ask. People like that.

One patient stands out in my mind. She was a lovely woman in her 80s who, early on, seemed sad much of the time. She stayed with us about four weeks. One of our nurses found out that this woman was at one time a well-known artist in our town. Our nurse teamed with a therapist and together they encouraged our patient to pick up a brush and paint again. Soon "Betty" (not her real name) was wheeling around in her wheelchair with paints, brush, and paper at the ready. You never knew where she might stop, pull out her brushes and go to work. Everyone begged for her paintings. Her family was beside themselves. Betty was her old self. Smiles everywhere! A team at work!

Being a dabbler at painting myself, I found Betty very intriguing. When discharged from our facility, she planned to go on a long train trip with her daughter and then start painting lessons for her great-granddaughter.

Betty's spirit was alive and well. I decided I would pay her a visit at home. I walked into her living room, where every bit of available wall space was testimony to Betty's artistic achievement. I was in awe. The long and the short of this story is that I wrote a half-page news article with photos of Betty and some of her art. I figured my article would be sliced and diced before it was published. There must have been a dearth of news that week, because my copy printed without one word changed and "guest columnist" written under my name. Betty and her family took pride in seeing her back in the news. And our physical rehab center had unlimited mileage in free press. All because a dedicated nurse and creative therapist worked together to make a difference for a patient. Teamwork. This you can market. And you must know that I proudly distributed copies of that article in many places.

A truly satisfying project that brings a smile to my face is the photo shoot we did to publicize our facility. After interviewing a few photographers, I selected one who I believed could do a good job for a reasonable price. Then the work began. Clipboard in hand, I walked the area, listing each potential shot. Next, I called former patients and my volunteer friends to be models. No one turned us down. All our staff at the unit and others in the hospital also agreed to participate. Once I had the complete list of people, I listed each shoot with all the characters and an approximate shoot time. A detailed list of what clothing each participant would need to have was also distributed. Before I could finalize all the times I had to be sure that I could secure the photo areas when I needed them—the gym, the activity room, an empty patient room, and so on. Since physicians, nursing staff, dietitians, social workers, and therapists were involved, there were many schedules to be coordinated. The common thread on the day of the shoot was flexibility, yet we stuck to our timetable well. I also had a photo release form ready for signing by each participant as we proceeded. (I decided that the next time we had a photo session, I'd get the photo release and a few other minor tasks completed before event day.)

I also organized a buffet lunch for everyone to make the occasion a little more fun and to allow for easy flow throughout the day. People could enjoy lunch at their convenience when not involved in the shoot. The camera rolled all day, loading and reloading color and black-and-white film. Our end product was more than 200 shots, composed of color slides and prints, as well as black-and-white pictures. We shot photos of a patient birthday party, group discussion, pet therapy, and therapists interacting with patients on each piece of gym equipment. We also captured activities of daily living, scenes with nurses and physicians, admissions, dietary, speech language pathologists with patients, and several other scenes. By the end of that day, I had a feeling of exhilarated exhaustion. Some of our former patients had traveled more than fifty miles to be part of the shoot. It was a great reunion and emotionally very rewarding.

The project enabled us to build slide presentations, photo boards, and albums that could be used everywhere in our marketplace. During hospital week, have a full set of black-and-white photos from which to choose the best compositions. Take several of the best photographs to accompany your prepared copy, and you have a premier press package. You are now ready to send these off to your local newspaper, well ahead of all your competitors. And for all your other events for which you need a photo and aren't able to take one, you have a great backup at the ready.

A professional video production is another excellent vehicle to consider in taking your program to the public. A well-prepared video document, coupled with a self-contained VCR/television system, makes a good tool for healthcare marketing. You can use this system before luncheons and meetings, as well as during open houses and various other events.

Health fairs for the community are everywhere. That does not mean you do not want to consider one. There are also several community events, such as Fourth of July celebrations, Memorial Day, fall fests, and senior events, to name a few. Offer to host a booth. If you can offer a health benefit with giveaways, you are in business. One of our best booths was "finger casting" for a local business with more than 500 employees. They held a health and craft fair for all employees and their families. The fair was in late October and we had a steady line all day with tots to teens getting slide-off finger casts to use for pre-Halloween fun. Our booth was a main attraction and we distributed and communicated a great deal of information about our facility that day. It cost very little, and we had lots of fun. The only downside was "pickled fingers" at the end of the day for anyone who had dipped and casted. On another day we helped a local business of about 200 people with their health fair. This time our theme was assisting with blood cholesterol tests. We supplied juice and muffins, using a few of our staff. The benefits received are still ongoing.

Marketing to the business community is also a vital link in marketing to the public. Try to look for what a business needs from you. In one community, drug screens were not being handled as efficiently as they should have been. It was the one recurring comment I heard as I asked businesses what they would like our hospital to offer. When first approaching department managers about the project, I saw eyes roll and heads turn in negative response. Persistence pays. We formed a team of department managers and packaged a program that was user-friendly to our customers. We did it—in spite of ourselves.

Many business enterprises and corporations just want presenters for brown-bag lunches. Large industries may have wellness centers and want medical support for their in-house health fairs. Without a doubt, many opportunities and challenges abound for us as innovative marketers.

The best advice is to use the following three tools:

1. Perseverance
2. Persistence
3. Tenacity

Earlier I mentioned lead time. I've noticed that people in marketing always have to run a little faster than anyone else. Deadlines are everywhere. If you are just starting, you will need to be fanatical about time lines. But always and forever make sure that you allow the time cushion. For example, if you truly need something done by June 13, then you ask for a deadline of June 8. Always plan for the unexpected. If you do not, you'll be sorry.

When you submit anything for print, never be the only one who proofreads. It takes a minimum of three sets of eyes.

In the beginning of this chapter I referred to planning. Planning is constant, never ending, and always changing. The key for me is to have a plan B in the wings. I have had to grab for plan B more than once.

For children, the gift of creativity flows endlessly. In marketing, we need to get back into our child's mind occasionally. *Find a way or make a way.*

13
CHAPTER

Developing Your Relationship with the Media

INTRODUCTION—by Sandy Lutz

The most difficult thing about working with the media on a story about the continuum of care is helping them with this simple question: "What the heck is it?" The term *continuum of care* sounds like something a journalist could rationally develop a definition for, but actually defining it is another matter.

Obviously, the first step in bridging this knowledge gap is helping the media understand the distinctive steps involved in a continuum of care. Healthcare clinicians and professionals often add to the confusion by using different terms for similar types of care. What's more, many forms of treatment overlap, adding even further to this confusing mix. We recommend that providers supply reporters and editors with a definition of treatment terms to help them understand all of this.

Few reporters are going to want to write a story on a subject that they don't understand or can't explain to their readers. And obviously, if they don't comprehend it, they're more likely to make a mistake. With the exception of some trade press, reporters aren't going to let sources read a story before it goes to press. That underscores the need to thoroughly brief reporters on what the continuum of care is and how it is relevant to their readers.

Most reporters can understand the difference between inpatient care and outpatient care. It's those gray areas in between that cause the most trouble. Subacute care, skilled nursing care, rehabilitation services, step-down units, long-term care—what are the differences? How do patients move from one setting to another? A question that a reporter is even more likely to ask is why a patient would go from one setting to another? A provider should expect such questions, and a media-savvy provider will be prepared with answers that neither confuse the reporter with jargon nor oversimplify the issue.

The reasons for different types of care in the course of treatment are determined by reimbursement, physicians' orders, patient preferences, and expected outcomes. All of these might be included in an explanation. However, an overemphasis on reimbursement might prompt questions about whether money or a patient's well-being are to account for the patient being moved from one setting to the next.

Providers know that insurers and government payors dictate the treatment pathway a patient might follow. However, it's wise not to start pointing fingers. Others—the payors, for example—may very well point them back at the provider, accusing them of trying to maximize reimbursement by keeping a patient in a higher-paying hospital unit.

Outcomes are an excellent context in which to talk about a continuum of care. With the recent emphasis on "report cards" for HMOs, more journalists will be likely to ask about outcomes and how different treatment settings and care from different types of healthcare professionals make a difference in a patient's care.

Certain physicians can be great interview subjects for reporters. However, it's important to make sure the physician has the time to deal with a reporter and the many questions he or she might have on this complex subject. Physicians are busy people and they can be difficult to get on the phone for an interview. This can be problematic if the reporter is using them as the main sources for a story. What's more, it can be an even bigger problem if the reporter has follow-up questions when writing the story a day or two later. However, if physicians are fairly accessible and aren't condescending with the media, they can be great interview subjects. Obviously, the physicians' orders control much of this process. That's why they can optimally explain how and why a patient would move through the continuum of care.

GETTING STARTED WITH THE MEDIA—by Janet Howe

As the saying goes, "You aren't who you think you are, but who your audience perceives you to be." Providing positive information about your facility to print and broadcast media in your market not only helps to enhance your reputation as a quality healthcare provider but also builds a bank of trust on which to draw should a crisis occur.

Reporters, editors, and program producers are people just like us—each appreciating the time you take to get to know them and to know the kinds of stories they are seeking for their publication or program. Personal contact is a must.

Meeting Your Local Media

Just as you make marketing calls to establish referral relationships, you also will need to contact local news media to create a network of communications. Here are some tips:

- Find out which reporters in your community's newspapers, magazines, and radio and television stations cover healthcare. Learn their names and titles, as well as the best times of day to call them.

- If you are new in your position, send a press release to these healthcare media to announce your arrival.

- Call and introduce yourself briefly. Reporters are always on deadline and appreciate your respect for that.

- Set up a lunch or dinner meeting if that is convenient to the reporter. Many media outlets have stringent rules about reporters accepting gifts and entertainment from potential news sources, so be sensitive about offering to pay for meals.

- When you meet, be sure to find out what kinds of stories interest the reporter, what the news deadlines are, whether the reporter likes to accept news tips and story ideas by phone, fax, letter, or manuscript.

TELLING YOUR STORY

- *Phone Calls:* Once you have established a relationship with a reporter, editor, or producer, you can call him or her with a brief story idea. Generally, the following are the best times to call:

Newspapers: Between 10 A.M. and 6 P.M. weekdays.

Television: Between 9 and 10 A.M. and after 4 P.M.

Magazines: Six to eight weeks in advance of the regularly scheduled publication date in the case of monthly or semimonthly publications; two weeks before delivery date if a weekly news magazine.

Radio: Times vary according to individual assignments. On weekends and after business hours, call for the assignments editor at print and electronic media.

■ *Press Release:* Send a press release to the media when you have hard news or a feature story about your facility. Be sure to first secure its approval from your facility's designated senior office. Remember that a press release must provide answers to the following questions: who, what, when, where, why, and how. Press releases must not contain opinion (opinions may be expressed through an editorial, letter to the editor, or a purchased "advertorial"). See *The Associated Press Stylebook* (available from AP and in bookstores) to make certain your release is written in paper journalistic style and to answer questions about punctuation, capitalization, and other rules.

■ *Follow-Up Contact:* If your press release has particular news value (not just an announcement), you may wish to call reporters and producers to determine their interest in your story.

■ *Story Ideas or Tip Sheets:* An additional way to keep your health-care facility's name in front of the media is periodically to send four or five brief story ideas (one paragraph, four to five sentences). They can be a continuation of an earlier press release or a health and safety tip from your clinical staff. These items are intended to interest the media in developing a feature story that may or may not have a particular time sensitivity.

■ *Press Conferences:* If you have a blockbuster story (such as a hospitalized VIP or a major clinical breakthrough), you may decide to call a press conference to tell your story at the same time to all media contacts. This avoids favoritism and provides your facility an opportunity to bring media on site. Again, be sure to clear this with your facility's designated senior officer.

■ *Newsletters:* If your facility publishes a newsletter that provides additional clinical or public service information, you may wish to send it to the media. If, however, your newsletter includes internal communications (staff information or directives that are proprietary to your facility), it should not be made available to the media.

KEEPING RECORDS AND MEASURING RESULTS

Three good ways to maintain your media program and to review its results include the following:

- *Mailing List:* Develop and regularly update your mailing list of media contacts. This may include local, regional, and national media as appropriate to your market. Check with your local public library or nearest chapter of the Public Relations Society of America or International Association of Business Communicators to determine what published media directories may be useful to you in reaching print and electronic media.

- *Media Inquiry Forms:* It's a good idea to record each of your media contacts on a media inquiry form (p. 163), noting the subject you discussed, with whom you discussed it, the date your contact was made, and the expected outcome of the inquiry. Later, you can refer to this record as you track results of your media relations program.

- *Press Clipping Service:* If you are in a large enough news market, you may wish to subscribe to a press clipping service that will monitor print media and clip articles mentioning your facility. This will let you know how much exposure you are getting and tell you when a local story may have been picked up by a wire service and reported across the country. Each time you send a press release, send a copy and its distribution list to the service so that they can watch for the story's appearance. Cost of the service generally is based on the number of clips you receive. Bacon's and Luce are two good clipping services.

MORE STRATEGIES

- *Press Breakfasts, Luncheons, or Dinners:* You may wish to include a few selected reporters each time you meet informally over a meal with your medical director or other key staff members. Have an agenda in mind, such as bringing reporters up to date on new therapies, new programs, new equipment, or other medical advances in your field.

- *Speakers Bureau/Media Experts List:* One of the best ways to build a positive media relationship is to position your facility and its staff as expert guest speakers in the community. Develop a list of experts and topics that they are qualified to discuss, then mail this with a cover letter to media as well as community, school, and religious organizations.
- *Photography/Graphics:* Ours is a visual culture. You will find that stories that can be illustrated are often more readily used by the media. When making a personnel announcement, be sure to include a small head shot of the subject. If suggesting a news feature, send along good snapshots or, if budget allows, professional photos of the item or event. In the case of clinical stories or stories on financial or demographic issues, you may wish to include clear medical illustrations or charts and graphs.

MEDIA CONTACT

Any contact between your facility and the media can have far-reaching consequences—positive or negative. To ensure a positive outcome it is important to have a procedure for handling media contact in place before contact occurs. We suggest making available to all employees a brief set of procedural instructions that they can refer to when necessary. Following is a model of such a sheet. You need only add the names of the appropriate officers in the spaces provided.

Incoming media inquiries should be first directed to your senior media relations officer and next to _____. No other staff member of the facility has the authority to respond to media inquiries. This is true both for disseminating news from the facility, as well as for answering incoming media contacts.

All outgoing contacts must be cleared by the _____.

All incoming media calls should be directed to the _____ and coordinated with the _____.

If a media call is received at night or on a weekend, the call should be directed to the _____ 's residence or to the residence of the _____ and to the _____ they will decide how best to respond to the inquiry.

The Role of the Media Contact

If you receive an inquiry from the media, it is important to remember the following:

■ *Keep Accurate Records:* Use your media inquiry form to keep accurate track of every inquiry received, how it was handled, and the outcome. This will be a valuable reference for the future. Be sure to note the date of the inquiry, who represented the media, any competitors who may have been used as resources, and so on.

■ *Obtain Information Thoroughly:* When answering a media inquiry, the most important thing to remember is that you are responsible for managing the news opportunity. Be helpful to the media, yet do not feel obligated to discuss topics about which you are not comfortable or knowledgeable. Honesty is the best policy in all cases. If you do not know the answer, tell the inquirer that you will have to check your resources and call him or her back. Be sure to keep your word and follow up in a timely manner.

Before you answer any questions, determine what the reporter specifically needs. Follow the format of your media inquiry form to obtain the following information:

■ *Vital Statistics:* Record the date and time of the call, name of the print or electronic communications, the caller's name and phone number, the information requested, and the deadline. Ask the reporter to specify questions so that you can enter them on the media inquiry form. This will help prepare for the subsequent media interview and determine the nature of the reporter's story. Also ask with whom the reporter has already spoken; this helps put the story into perspective.

■ *Angle of the Story:* Determine whether this story has a local angle or whether it is regional or national in scope.

■ *Nature of the Story:* Determine if your facility is an appropriate resource, or if the reporter is attempting to draw your facility into a controversial issue.

■ *Who the Other Story Sources Are:* Ask who else is being quoted in this story. This will help you determine if it is appropriate for your facility to be quoted in this story.

■ *Who Is Needed for an Interview:* Asking this question will help you determine if the reporter needs to speak with a management source or a clinical source. After hearing the nature of the story, you may decide that the requested person is not the appropriate source for this subject and choose to direct the reporter to another resource within your facility.

After obtaining the information you need, you can take the following actions:

■ Decide if your facility should respond to the media inquiry or if the reporter should be directed to outside industry sources, such as a national association for your specialty.

■ Tell the reporter that you must verify some of the answers to his or her questions and that you will call back. Be sensitive to the reporter's deadline and respect it by keeping your word. If you know you will not be able to meet this deadline, say so up front and offer a more reasonable time.

■ If appropriate, set an appointment for the reporter to interview the appropriate unit resource.

■ Develop answers to possible media questions. Then sit in on the interview to take detailed notes or to tape record if appropriate and with the consent of the reporter.

To get more information, try the following:

■ Refer to "Tips for Working with the Media" on p. 154.

■ Ask the reporter for all of the information required by your media inquiry form. They expect and are usually prepared to handle your questions. Be sure to record their answers on your inquiry form so that you have a record of the call and begin to get a sense of individual reporters and the needs of their news organizations.

■ For inquiries on specific patients, see "Release of Patient Information" on p. 159.

■ For inquiries on specific patients, see "Release of Confidential Information" on Page 160.

■ For interviews that require filming or photographing of patients, see "Photographing/Filming Patients" on p. 161.

CRISIS COMMUNICATIONS

A crisis situation is a decisive moment, a turning point, and may include such instances as natural disasters, admission of a public figure to the unit, legal action, a major financial or administrative action, or crime.

A crisis need not be negative or result in negative media coverage. Remember that, to a degree, how you handle responses to the media will affect the outcome of reporting. By demonstrating willingness to cooperate with media inquiries and answering questions with an honest, proactive intention, you may capture the opportunity to gain the respect and support of the media and your community.

Following are media policies that must be followed in a crisis.

Notification of Appropriate Parties

If you anticipate a media crisis or are contacted by the media about a potentially negative circumstance, proper handling of the situation is imperative. Contacts from national news media on issues with national ramifications—positive or negative—as well as local contacts regarding crisis issues must be handled through the appropriate officer.

Designating a Spokesperson

After notifying and engaging appropriate parties, the next action is to name a spokesperson to represent the hospital. The executive director is generally the designated media spokesperson for a hospital. This individual is responsible for choosing a backup person (usually the marketing director) in case the executive director is unavailable to respond to a media inquiry. Once a spokesperson is selected, continue to use the same person throughout the crisis.

The executive director and his or her designated backup are the *only* people authorized to answer questions from the media on behalf of the hospital. Advise all staff of this policy because it is important to limit who in the hospital communicates with the media.

Directions for the Specialty Program Spokesperson

- Enter into an interview only after thorough preparation (development of anticipated questions and answers and exhaustive review of the facts). Have your marketing director prepare background on current events that might prompt the reporter to expand the line of questioning on this story.
- Before the interview, select and prepare an ad hoc committee of hospital personnel (such as the marketing director, medical director, and unit program director) to conduct fact finding and to assist in developing responses to media inquiries.
- Gather facts to support your response, taking this opportunity to guide the interview with positive information about your facility.
- Rehearse your answers to questions and the delivery of your message until you are comfortable with the content and able to communicate succinctly, positively, and confidently.
- Keep your marketing director and other key staff informed. If the crisis lasts for more than one day, ask the marketing director to handle calls by reading a brief, agreed-upon statement.

- These statements should be updated daily or, depending upon the nature of the crisis, twice daily. Good times to deliver updates are 10 A.M. and 4 P.M. daily.
- If the issue has legal implications, have statements cleared by the hospital's corporate legal counsel.
- Alert your personnel not to become involved in discussions with reporters.
- Keep all appropriate staff briefed on a daily basis. Remember that the media are not your only audience.

Role of the Specialty Program Medical Director

The medical director may be called upon by executive director to comment on special issues or respond to media inquiries involving clinical issues. Direct response to the media by the medical director should be done so only at the executive director's request.

Role of Hospital Marketing Director

- Prepare the executive director or other appointed spokesperson as you would for any media interview. Anticipate questions and help him or her prepare answers to them.
- Coordinate and screen press calls. Make sure that all calls related to the crisis come through your office—not to the executive director or the director's assistant. Failure to coordinate calls and direct them through one source can result in confusion and increase the chance that calls will not be answered appropriately or promptly.
- Plan your strategy. With the executive director, decide if the situation will be best handled by holding a press conference, a press briefing, or through individual interviews.
- If this crisis is expected to last for several days and/or has attracted a number of media, you will need to develop an immediate action plan that may include a combination of strategies.
- Prepare a written statement, agreed upon by your executive director, and use it to respond to all media inquiries. Update this statement with short news bulletins twice daily (10 A.M. and 4 P.M. are good times). Announce at the time of one bulletin when the next one will be given. The more information you include in a statement, the more you will satisfy the media and the easier your job will be.

- If the situation is best handled by a one-time news conference, prepare the executive director accordingly. Although time will probably be short, be prepared with as many visuals as possible to clarify the issues (charts, large graphics, videotapes, press kits, etc.).

- Keep good records. Document all statements; use the media inquiry forms to keep an accurate log of press inquiries and your responses.

- Act as a spokesperson. You may be able to serve as a more neutral voice than the executive director. When a statement has to be extremely brief (as in a situation with legal implications), it may come best from the marketing director.

- Screen calls. The marketing director, not the executive director or his or her assistant, should screen calls and arrange press conferences if approved by the executive director.

Media Crisis Kits

In planning ahead for crisis communications, be sure to have all necessary information you will need at hand at all times. Ahead of time, prepare a portfolio that includes:

- Copies of the policy guide
- Copies of patient permission forms
- Copies of media inquiry forms
- A roster of key office and home phone numbers for facility personnel (executive director, director of marketing, medical director, chief financial officer)

Provide a kit to each of the following:

- Executive director
- Administrator on call
- Marketing director
- Marketing staff
- Risk manager
- Evening director of nursing

These kits should be kept at home and referred to in case a crisis occurs after hours. The evening supervisor of nursing will want to keep the kit at his or her desk.

MEDIA ISSUES WITH LEGAL IMPLICATIONS

All potential comments to the media on issues with potential legal implications must first be reviewed by the executive director and the facility's general counsel. Possible comments must also be reviewed with the appropriate parties before any discussion with the media.

Following is a sample set of procedural instructions that you might want to post for the benefit of the employees at your facility. Simply add the appropriate names and phone numbers as indicated.

- For facility issues related to risk management (such as patient or visitor injuries and potential resulting lawsuits against the hospital, call:

    (Name of insurance company)
    (24-hour phone number): _____
    (Name of on-call attorney)

- For all other legal issues (such as employee arrests, breach of contract, etc.) with potential for resulting in lawsuits against the hospital, call:

    (General Counsel)
    (Facility)
    Work phone: _____
    Home phone: _____

TIPS FOR WORKING WITH THE MEDIA

These tips apply to both crisis and routine situations. Feel free to copy this section from the media relations guide and share it with those who have permission to speak to the media.

1. Direct media calls to the director of marketing. Either transfer the call to marketing or take the reporter's name, the name of the publication, and the phone number, and alert the marketing office immediately.

2. Don't avoid the press. Return phone calls from reporters as soon as possible, preferably within the hour. The more helpful you are to the press, the more you earn their respect and balanced attention. It is better to be candid than to say "no comment" or to be unreachable. (Any of these actions imply you have something to hide.) In this manner you may avoid one-sided stories.

3. Provide information promptly when a reporter calls, but avoid incomplete answers. If you need time to check your sources, tell the reporter you will call him or her right back. Then respond promptly.

4. Use short, direct words as often as possible. Your quotes will be more usable and accurate. If you are concerned about being misquoted, say so. Ask the reporter's cooperation. Most reporters understand you can't say everything about the situation for publication.

5. Always tell the truth. Your credibility and the credibility of your unit and the facility are at stake.

6. Be factual when you answer questions. Avoid long-winded explanations of why your program or facility is the best unless you have supporting documentation.

7. Never offer personal opinions when speaking on behalf of your facility. If you are asked for and agree to give a personal opinion, make certain the reporter understands you are speaking for yourself and are not presenting the views of your facility.

8. Comment only on matters within your area of expertise. Sometimes a reporter may ask you to comment on a related subject or controversial issue and promise not to use your name. Unless you know the reporter well and trust him or her, you should decline such requests.

9. Repeat important points you wish to make when talking with print reporters. Speak slowly and spell difficult words and names. Repeat figures, and if they are critical, ask the reporter to repeat them to you.

10. Have a succinct printed version of your statement available when you are interviewed. If you will be discussing a difficult subject and are concerned about the reporter getting the facts straight, a written statement can help clarify the situation.

11. Avoid going off the record. Most reporters do not like it because they would rather use a quotable source. Also, it is really a gentleman's agreement between you and the reporter. Unfortunately, not all reporters are ladies or gentlemen. If for some reason, however, you feel that you

must make remarks off the record, use the following standards of journalistic ethics:

- Preface each statement by saying, "The following is off the record."
- Indicate clearly when you are on the record again.
- Don't say belatedly, "The material I have just given you is off the record."

12. Don't assume the reporter understands the healthcare field. Medical/health reporters are often very bright; however, a general reporter or an inexperienced reporter will sometimes pretend to know what you are talking about rather than admit ignorance or confusion. Seek feedback from the reporters to determine their interpretation of what you have said.

13. Do not ask to see the reporter's copy before it is published or broadcast. The reporter is under no obligation to show copy. If scientific or technical data is involved, you might suggest that the reporter check back with you for accuracy on your portion of the story. The reporter often will appreciate your offering to check accuracy.

14. Don't let the reporter put words in your mouth. Some reporters will try to manipulate what you say by restating your comments: "So in other words . . . ." Keep control of the interview by rephrasing the questions if necessary.

15. If a serious error appears in print, ask to have it corrected. The marketing director should handle errors in print. Decide whether or not an error is worth correcting or is correctable. If it is serious and it is not corrected, it may be repeated both in the original and in other publications. If satisfaction cannot be obtained from the reporter, then a joint decision by the executive director and marketing director should be made to call or write a letter to the editor.

16. Timeliness is essential when sending letters to the editor. If a letter to the editor is the best route (whether it is related to your article or to any article), don't wait more than a week to respond. It will no longer be considered news if you wait longer.

Special Guidelines for Working with Broadcast Media

1. When contacted by a radio station, remember that your comments may be taped. A radio reporter will often tape you over the phone, sometimes without your permission. Do not be caught off guard. Ask reporters if you are being taped and gain their specific questions before agreeing to a taped interview. If you would like to think about and formulate answers to the questions, tell the reporter you will return the call at an agreed-upon time.

2. Remember the following appearance tips when preparing for television interviews, whether taped or live:

   - You are representing your facility; a well-groomed appearance is essential.

   - Wear what you would normally wear for the setting. For example, if you are taped in your laboratory, office, or clinical setting, and a white coat or uniform is part of that setting, then wear it. Otherwise, normal office attire is appropriate. Normal office attire also is appropriate if you are going to the station to be interviewed. If for some reason you are taped at your home, more casual attire is acceptable.

   - Unless you are on a talk show, you are usually seen only from the waist up. Because the camera focuses on your head, remember to check your hair. Other distractions are crooked ties, collars, and jackets. Make sure your attire is straight.

   - If you are being interviewed at your facility, use camera crew setup time to ask the reporter questions about the structure of the interview, and use this as an opportunity to summarize what you wish to discuss.

3. During a television interview:

   - Look at the reporter, not at the camera. Relax; don't fidget. At the end of a taped interview, the reporter may reask certain questions, asking for shortened answers, while the cameraperson tapes you from the opposite direction. These are called "reversals" and are needed for editing purposes. They also tape "listening shots" when no sound is being recorded.

- If you wish to say something off camera, ask if the sound or the tape recorder is on. Remember that television reporters usually have a tape recorder with them as well as the camera and sound equipment.

- Be brief. The average recorded quote in a broadcast news story runs under thirty seconds. You must expect your responses to be edited; broadcast media like to use sound bites, which are quotable, brief sections of an interview that capture the essence of the story. The shorter your answers, the less editing your remarks will receive.

4. Anticipate questions and develop answers that state your key ideas clearly and succinctly. Avoid complicated and time-consuming answers.

FINAL POINTS TO REMEMBER

Once you have established good working relationships with the media, do not negate your efforts by playing favorites. If there is a major piece of news occurring at your hospital, make sure to share it with all of the appropriate press members. It is important to develop a reputation for fairness when working with members of the press. Let reporters know, through a brief phone call or letter, when they have written or broadcast a well-balanced story. Reporters are human and appreciate positive feedback.

Following are several forms and sets of guidelines that deal with communications with the media. They can be consulted as various media situations arise.

RELEASE OF PATIENT INFORMATION

Release of Nonconfidential Information

The following nonconfidential information may be released for all patients *without* the patient's authorization.

1. Patient's name.
2. The fact that an individual is a patient at your facility.
3. The patient's condition at the time of inquiry. The following terms shall be used to describe a patient's condition (this information is to be determined by the physician or the charge nurse):

GOOD   Vital signs are stable and within normal limits. Patient is conscious and comfortable; prognosis is favorable.

FAIR   Vital signs are stable and within normal limits. Patient is conscious but may be uncomfortable; prognosis is favorable.

SERIOUS   Vital signs may be unstable and outside normal limits. Patient is acutely ill; prognosis is questionable.

CRITICAL   Vital signs are unstable and outside normal limits. Patient may be unconscious; prognosis is unfavorable.

Adapted from American Hospital Association Guidelines.

RELEASE OF CONFIDENTIAL INFORMATION

For press inquiries about confidential information, the following rules apply:

1. If the patient is conscious and can communicate with the doctor or nurse in charge, he or she shall be asked whether she or he will permit any further information other than name and condition to be released (such as the nature of the illness or injury). The patient's decision is final. (Use the authorization for publication form included on p. 162.)
2. For minors under 18 years of age, the parent's or legal guardian's consent is required.
3. If the patient is unconscious or unable to communicate, the decision must be made by next of kin.

Death of a Hospital Patient

1. News of the death of a hospital patient becomes public *after* the family has been notified.
2. Information on the cause of death must come from the patient's physician, and its release must be approved by family members.
3. The name of the mortuary receiving the body may be released to the press.

PHOTOGRAPHING/FILMING PATIENTS

When the media requests to film or photograph a patient, the following rules shall apply:

1. Pictures of patients are to be taken only with the permission of the patient or next of kin.

2. No pictures of unconscious patients will be taken.

3. For minors under 18 years of age, the permission of a parent or legal guardian is required.

4. Patients agreeing to photographs or videotaping must sign an authorization for publication form (see p. 162). The marketing director should keep blank forms in his or her office. After the form is signed, it should be returned to the marketing director's office to be filed for the record. File a separate, signed form for each event.

Adapted from Amercian Hospital Association Guidelines.

AUTHORIZATION FOR PUBLICATION

(NAME OF FACILITY)

(This form is only for use with media interviews, videotaping, and photography involving patients or employees.)

I, _____, do hereby authorize
                    (Full Name)

_____, to disclose information for publication

or electronic viewing, other than advertising, concerning my or my

child's, _____, medical care.
                    (Full Name)

I also authorize _____ and/or the news
                                (Full Name)

media to photograph, videotape and/or record me or my child,

_____, for publication or electronic viewing,
            (Full Name)

other than advertising, while a patient at _____.
                                                    (Facility Name)

I release the facility, its physicians, employees, and consultants from any liability in connection with the use of such materials.

                                                    Signed:

_____
            Date
                                        _____
                                                    Name

                                        _____
                                                    Address

_____
            Witness
                                        _____
                                                    City, State

Please return completed form to: Indicate which of the following
Director of Marketing of   has signed:

                                        ❏ Patient
_____   ❏ Parent or Guardian of Patient
            Facility Name   ❏ Employee

MEDIA INQUIRY FORM

Date: _____ Time: _____

Requested by (radio, TV, newspaper, wire service, magazine): _____

_____

_____

Editor/Producer: _____ Reporter/Host: _____

Phone: _____

Nature of call: _____

_____

_____

_____

Date Information Needed: _____

Action Taken: _____

_____

_____

_____

Results and Evaluation: _____

_____

_____

Person Receiving Inquiry: _____

Notes: _____

_____

_____

Marketing to Physicians

In specialty service marketing, the primary targets are physicians. We often use the phrase, "While anyone may initiate a referral, admission is by physician order." Marketers must develop a complete strategy to market to all levels of census builders: immediate census builders (hospital-based discharge-planning professionals, nurses, and other healthcare professionals), intermediate census builders (physicians and physician office staff), and long-term census builders (the public, managed care, etc). We may concentrate our efforts in other areas, as noted in earlier chapters, so that efforts are complete. However, without the support of physicians, programs will not be successful. Many of the techniques used in marketing to physicians are traditional sales approaches such as one-to-one office visits and luncheons. This chapter will focus on the research and strategy in planning the physician marketing effort. Physician marketing techniques are consistent throughout the continuum, although the individual products and promotional tools vary.

BEFORE YOU GO—WHAT YOU SHOULD KNOW

When you first begin to develop your physician target list, the tendency is to go to the physicians who seem the nicest or those who are seen often in the facility. This is not necessarily the right way to proceed, because they may offer no referral potential. We recommend that you collect as much research as possible regarding physicians.

First, stop at the management information systems (MIS) department. In a hospital setting this may mean going to the actual department, but within a single provider setting this may be as simple as going to the clerical staff to generate a list of all the physicians who have either actively referred or those who have been the physician of a patient who was referred by another healthcare professional. The sorting of material can be done in a myriad of ways so that a profile of the practice is generated. (The profile may not be a totally accurate picture of the practice. We will address that later.) Basically, you are interested in such information as the type of patients referred, diagnoses, payor mix, and length of stay or treatment regimen ordered. If there is access to the hospital admit information or Med Par data this may reveal additional opportunities for referrals through additional education.

A visit to the medical staff offices of hospitals will often provide a guide to the medical staff. Many hospitals now produce glossy booklets with information about and photos of the medical staffs. This information usually includes where the physician attended medical school and completed residency and board certification. Even if one is not a hospital-based marketer, this is an excellent way to get the information needed, especially because of the pictures. If you happen to be good with names and faces (and believe me, this is a skill that marketers should cultivate), you can study these booklets so that you can introduce yourself to physicians in the hallways of facilities and make their acquaintance. It isn't always just celebrities who are flattered to be recognized. Besides, if they did not want to be recognized they never would have gone to the photo session.

Talk to the staff members of your facility, program, or provider. If they have experience with a physician, be it positive or negative, you simply must have this information before you walk out of the door. Take it from someone who has been there: There is no greater disservice to yourself as a marketer than to ignore opportunities to collect information that is virtually at your fingertips. Your staff is aware if the physician has referred or has not referred. They are aware of problems with the physician or patients. As you can imagine, having this information before a visit could be helpful.

If your program has patient satisfaction surveys, review those to determine if the physician's patients have been happy with the program. As we have mentioned in Chapter 20, "The Marketer's Toolbox," using the patient satisfaction survey can be an excellent tool in working with physicians to review their patients' perceptions and address issues and successes.

Know Your Product

Many people believe that the most successful marketer for specialty programs is a clinician. I prefer to think that the most successful marketer is a believer. If you believe in the product because you know someone who benefited, you will promote with a passion. That is one reason why it is so important to become thoroughly educated on the product or program before making the first call. How can one accomplish this? Shadow the professionals delivering care and ask questions. Ask for reference materials to read. Talk to families and patients to see what they have to say about the treatment. You don't have to be clinical, although it helps. One individual who participated in this book has a nonclinical background but has spent the last two years taking courses at night in anatomy, physiology, and biology so that she is more familiar with clinical areas. She was concerned that she did not have enough credibility for working with physicians. It is always good to broaden one's knowledge base but remember that no one can know all the ins and outs of a program and all of the different types of patients seen, or every potential variation or response to treatment. It is much more important to balance information with the ability to say, "I don't have the answer to that question, but I will get back to you with it." This is an opportunity to demonstrate consideration for the referral source's questions, show follow-up and commitment to the relationship, and most of all, to learn.

Remember that two heads are better than one—take someone with you. No one can answer questions or address misconceptions better than someone in authority within the program who has the power to change things in response to a physician's needs. If in the past there was an issue with reports, take the program director to acknowledge the past problem and share how the service is improving this situation. Department managers and program directors can successfully promote their own continuum services because they have day-to-day responsibility for their operations. This is especially important in addressing misconceptions that may exist. No one can more effectively address these than the individual in charge of the service. The marketers' credibility is at stake every time he or she walks into a physician's office. Taking an individual who actually can address issues and resolve them is a great strategy.

CASE STUDY

One of the interviewees for this book works a great deal with physicians to resolve issues. One of the areas in which physicians had concerns regarding her facility was with the scheduling department. She made appointments with physicians. The department director accompanied her on calls to address issues directly and share the intricacies of the department. Soon some of the offices were commenting that they mostly interacted with a certain member of the scheduling team and that they didn't have a face to go with a name. The marketer then matched up the individual schedulers with the offices that they generally contacted and made a point to take them on calls so they could introduce themselves. Now that the office staff and physicians have a bond with the personnel, they address issues as they arise and have established a more mutually beneficial relationship. The interviewee said that there were many naysayers who told her that this could cost the facility time, but she stressed that in the long run it was building relationships with the facility as a whole that would ensure the facility's success. She emphasizes that relationship-building does not occur overnight, and the focus is to promote the facility and the continuum in its entirety.

THE FIRST CONTACT

The first contact with a physician's office is to quantify and qualify the physician, that is, whether the physician should be placed on the marketer's target list and eventual rotation schedule. This is a relatively easy and painless visit. For maximum use of time, consider making this visit a get-to-know-you call only on the practice manager, nurse, or member of the office staff. These individuals can assist in efforts to qualify the physician. Refer to the physician profile form at the end of this chapter. You will note that inquiry into the medical background is prominent on the form. Next is information about the practice. Our mission here is to determine specifics. I usually start out with the practice manager or another key individual by stating that I am aware that they know all the specifics about the practice, and I hope they will tell me a little about it—what types of patients they see, and so on. This lead-in question usually generates a great deal of information and provides the opportunity to ask more specific questions. Payor mix is a touchy subject for many persons. There are skilled marketers who shy away from asking this question. There is an effective way to get this information. I usually notice the managed care and insurance provider cards or stickers at the reception window. I ask if they see a lot of managed care or insurance patients, then ask about how many, or what percentage. Then I can mention that I have heard payors can be difficult to work with and ask who they work with the most or who they like working with the most. Usually this offers the opportunity to probe deeper. If there are older patients seen in the office, I ask about Medicare, or if there are none, I comment on it. Either way, the office manager will usually volunteer the information. If the area is industrialized and the office population and specialty indicates, ask about workers' compensation. Based on this encounter, one can determine if return visits are indicated and approximately how often they are needed. I always follow these visits with handwritten thank-you notes that I usually write while still in my car in the parking lot. If I have scheduled a visit with the physician or a return visit for staff members, I am certain to include this in the notes. Keep in mind that handwritten thank-you cards marked personal will more likely get to the physician's desk than a letter on letterhead in a facility envelope.

One of our interviewees suggested that she has been most successful when she has targeted practices and offered to introduce herself over lunch. She emphasizes that most offices stop for lunch; it is just a question of when they stop. She says this method is less about sales than it is about building relationships and includes the staff who then get to know *her*, not just another vendor. She states that she has never been turned down when she has offered to take the staff lunch. This interviewee believes that many physicians are simply bombarded with materials and that the direct approach of leaving handouts such as program and Medicare coverage information for them to distribute to patients is much more effective. She calls offices to set up appointments; she never uses cold calls. "Cold calls can result in cold shoulders, and office staff seem to appreciate respect for their time," she said.

If you are part of an organization, share the information you have gathered at the facility's marketing meeting. With the advent of more aggressive marketing, some well-meaning facilities have turned loose large marketing forces on their physicians and do not stop to consider that they all are collecting the same information. Just think how irritating it would be to have multiple individuals calling on you all asking the same question. Share the information. This introduces another problem. As we have developed multiple marketing staffs, many part of their own cost-based unit personnel, we have invited crossover and have harrassed the medical staffs. You would be surprised at how many times I have made calls and been told that another person from the organization was just here yesterday. "Don't you people talk to each other?" they ask. One physician angrily pointed out to me that he sees the hospital reps because he feels that he should and genuinely wants to be knowledgeable, but resents that no one seems to care that he has a business to run and patients to see. He stated that if he wasn't seeing multiple reps from the same provider at different times he would be able to see patients more efficiently. Obviously, this is a legitimate complaint—one which we have created. The solution, again, is to cross-train marketing reps and centrally manage the entire contact effort.

CROSS-FUNCTION, NOT CROSS-PURPOSES

If we have so indoctrinated our staffs that they are focused on one goal—their individual program census—that they do not see the big picture, then we have again disabled the continuum of care. One of the most difficult tasks marketing directors face is how to disseminate the marketing message with the most knowledgeable people delivering it. As continuums expand, the issue is not always how to market it but who should market it. Consider a healthcare organization with multiple continuum services. All too often there is one individual who prescreens (financially and physically) the referred patients in call program. This means that in a hospital referring an individual patient to rehab, skilled/subacute, or geropsych services, three different program reps may all go to the same person and conduct a screening. These same three people will all get back to both the physician and the discharge planning professional regarding the qualifications of the patient. If all three report approvals (and this actually could happen), then the decision may not be based on clinical appropriateness but on who had the best relationship or timing with the physician, discharge planning professional, or patient.

At the least, this is an inefficient system from our staff management standpoint and incredibly irritating and confusing (to some extent) to our physician staff, whom we are most likely trying to educate on at least one of the new programs. It is easy to see that we have created our own monster.

We have observed marketing directors dividing up the physician staff and giving directives that no crossover occur but never ensuring that exceptional cross education is in place. Others have given directives that teams go out to market. This team concept of marketing can be offputting; many classic sales trainers would recommend against it. We believe it is up to your team's capabilities, but we do not recommend sending more than two persons together. The key to success is the ability to listen and sell what the physician is interested in or to develop an area based on the types of patients seen. To do that, some level of cross education must occur.

Unfortunately, there is no right and perfect approach to managing the sales of the continuum. But we offer the following suggestions:

- All reps should be cross educated in continuum services to answer questions and to appropriately route leads to others.
- As part of sales training, teach the reps to listen and sell appropriately.
- Remove the fear of not selling an individual program by focusing on promoting the continuum; fear of losing one's job can be counterproductive.
- Remember that if a rep is truly successful, he or she has built a relationship and may be quite possessive of it. This becomes a proprietary issue if the territory or accounts are reassigned.

BUILDING A ROTATION SCHEDULE

At this point one will have qualified and quantified the physician and possess a list of who should and should not be seen. Don't be afraid to remove names from the list. The sales axiom of "80 percent of the business comes from 20 percent of the customers" should direct you to take off names and concentrate first on the most likely targets. Later, as the business base is solidified, there will be ample opportunity to add in the names of more targets that could be a rewarding challenge. Now it is time to prioritize the list to work more efficiently. This list will always be in some state of flux as new physicians move into the area and others leave or retire. An unchanging marketer's list should be a red flag in sales management.

The goal here is to plan and implement the physician-marketing effort to ensure increased patient flow as much as possible. Our focus is to alleviate swings in census and improve the conversion rate. Alleviating the dramatic swings in census can affect the entire delivery system by facilitating staffing planning. Improving the conversion rate means that we are working smarter, not harder, in converting more of our referrals instead of running around in a panic attempting to get more and more referrals.

For maximum benefit we suggest incorporating a tiered strategy to the physician-marketing effort based on the information gathered during one-to-one direct educational contacts. Consider an "A" list with highest potential and a "B" list with lesser potential.

We recommend physicians and their offices on Tier A be visited once every two weeks. (Remember this will hopefully be to deliver reports, patient satisfaction surveys, case studies, and so on.) This should shortly change to visits once a month to maintain the relationship. If referrals result there will be opportunity to visit informally often to deliver patient information. Physicians on Tier B should be visited twice in the first four to six weeks and once every six weeks thereafter. Again, if referrals result there will be opportunities to drop in with patient information. If an office happens to be literally in the neighborhood, it may be worthwhile to stop in and say hello.

This list of contacts that any rep will develop refers to office contacts. It does not necessarily reflect a physician in one-to-one contact on every visit. These visits are opportunities to deliver discharge reports, brochures, and so on and to build referral relationships. Make no mistake: The greatest referral sources are those with a solid relationship of trust and respect as a foundation. This does not occur overnight, just as friendships in our life do not occur overnight. This adds to the complexity of managing the multiple program reps. There is no accounting for how personalities mesh. The goal is to convey knowledge and promote referrals. Some reps are inherently more successful with certain physicians than others, and we must be flexible enough to change assignments and manage the perceived threat to another program rep. As reps we must be confident enough to suggest that another individual take over the account for the benefit of the continuum. As management we should see this as a victory and not an admission of poor performance.

Physicians' office staffs are traditionally recognized as gate-keepers. Consider including one-to-one educational contacts, brochures delivered to offices, and luncheon educational programs as strategies to develop referrals. These groups have been ignored in the past by some reps and the opportunity may exist to bring them into the fold with special events. One rep has told us about their "DOSE" group. A DOSE (doctor's office staff event) is held quarterly at a local hotel. Educational presentations are made over lunch, and door prizes are distributed. The events are well attended and have produced an increase in referrals for many of the hospital's services. The reps deliver flyers to physician offices; the office staff members call to RSVP.

SETTING REALISTIC GOALS

Unfortunately, when we go out to make calls on potential referral sources, we often set ourselves up for failure. Many of us tend to be optimistic, to believe that at the end of the day we will have a brief-case full of referrals. That is simply not the case. Encourage your team to set realistic goals when they go out. A friend of mine explains it this way: "There are only three reasons to go out. One is to overcome objections. One is to get a referral. And the most important one is to invent a reason to return." Needless to say when we first did training together, I looked at her with utter awe when she made this statement. When I conduct sales training now, I use her statement to prepare reps for the realities of sales calls. Direct care providers did not go into healthcare to do sales, we entered the field to help people. Many of us would say that clinical professionals are the best individuals to present clinical programs; however, those direct care providers sometimes equate sales as plaid jackets pushing defective used vehicles with a smile. It is important to not only train well but also to manage expectations. Encourage people just to look for a reason to return. This can be to deliver the materials you actually have in your portfolio during the call (remember, a reason to return the next day and demonstrate your follow-up) or to see the physician. We train people always to end their call by saying, "Is there anything I can help you with today?" While this is helpful and asks for the business, it is seldom perceived as insulting. Don't ever tell the team that referrals are out of the question.

CASE STUDY

I was conducting sales training for a new program rep in a hospital. He was a very bright young man and had just completed his degree in social work. This was his first job and he had taken the community rep position because nothing was available in the area in social work. He had expressed such trepidation and hesitation regarding sales that I had gone out of my way to reassure him by saying repeatedly, "Just think about a reason to return." I obviously went overboard because when he returned from his call, I asked about the visit and he stated that he had a reason to return. I congratulated his success on the call and was eager to give him confidence about his newly developing skills. I then asked him what was his reason to return. He gave a very sheepish grin and told me it would be to tell the physician whether or not we would accept the two referred patients he just asked us to screen. We both burst out laughing and I shook his hand and congratulated him. From that time on I used this as a success story during many company marketing sessions and he basked in the limelight of success. The moral of the story is to be sure to manage expectations, and hope the sky is the limit.

CONSIDER THE WORST MARKETING CALL A LEARNING EXPERIENCE

While experiences like that of the young man described above are wonderful, they are rare. Though we have calls that go down into our own personal call hall of fame, unfortunately we all will have calls that go very, very wrong, the type of calls that make us wonder what we are doing here. These calls have become a part of my sales training. The absolute worst one was on a physician. Our staffs need to understand that this is just a job and that in making calls no one will throw tomatoes at us or physically hurt us. But on days that you are looking for referrals and get none, a bad call can ruin a day. Many times these calls can be our own fault, such as when we do not do our homework before we go.

CASE STUDY

It was my very first job as a marketing director in an acute rehab hospital. I was ecstatic when I was given a note that said that Dr. So and So's office had called and wanted brochures. I packed up all of my promotionals (first mistake) and beelined over to the physician's office. (Keep in mind that I was new and really had not mastered listening and interpreting body language, lest you think I was just terminally dense!) Dr. So and So's office staff seemed very surprised to see me when I explained that someone had called and asked for brochures. No one had called, they assured me. Still, I kept insisting that Dr. So and So wanted these brochures. I gave out all my goodies and they agreed that they would tell the physician that I was here. Well, he came to the hall and I was ushered in. Imagine my surprise when he told me that not only did he not call, but that he would never call, because some of the physicians in the joint venture group were the same ones that had thoroughly blocked him from developing his new practice when he had finished his residency and moved here. He would not do "anything that would help the people who had tried to run him out of business." At this point, I was hoping a hole would open up to swallow me. I must have learned something in those sales training courses because I pointed out that I was certain that he cared about his patients above everything else and that my father had been a stroke victim who received no rehab care. I stated that if I could ever help him I would personally come over to screen the patient. He calmed down and talked about his patients and that they did come first. Even though we parted on better terms, I never saw one of his patients and we were the only facility within fifty miles. When I got back to the hospital, I tried to find out who took the message because it wasn't signed. I still don't know who wrote it. But to this day I feel certain that they knew the practice better than I did.

WHAT DO PHYSICIANS WANT?
Knowledge of the Best Care Available and All of the Options

I do believe that physicians want to take care of their patients and want them to have the best care possible. They truly do want knowledge, and probably nowhere is there a more successful example than their relationship with the pharmaceutical industry. With running a practice and trying to respond to the ever-changing healthcare system, what physician has time to read everything about every new drug that hits the market? The pharmaceutical industry responded to a need by providing reps to go to the physician's office and provide information and samples of the new drugs. It was an effective use of a physician's time to see the rep, and relationships were built. This same technique has been used by different industries such as in new equipment, home infusion, and home health. The information is valuable, but now there is much more competition for the physician's ear.

Ease of Access

Follow the same theory as above. In a nutshell, it is: "I am very busy, please make this easy." Have we explained the referral process, provided preprinted outpatient prescription pads, and so on? It has to be incredibly easy not only to refer but also to work with the provider on an ongoing basis. Take an honest hard look at your program. Is it user-friendly? Do you go to offices or homes to screen patients quickly? Do you get answers back in a timely fashion? Do you provide reports on patient progress? Or do you throw up barriers to access and smooth relationships, such as inflexible admitting or service hours, or excessive paperwork? Do you have a phone service that is so overloaded that the potential referral sources get busy signals? Ask your referral sources about their perceptions. You may be surprised. If you make it easy, however, you will promote referrals.

Quality Providers

While in one of my previous employer's corporations, the mandate was "quality is a given," we all know that it is not. Providers without accreditations or those with poor surveys will not likely come first on referrals for risk-management issues. What this means to those in good stead is: promote, promote, promote! If you have accreditations, do you reference this in program collaterals? Have you purchased accreditation stickers to affix to brochures and program communications? Did you publicize superior surveys or commendations? Have you made it as risk free as possible to refer? Something as simple as delivering patient-satisfaction surveys or sharing outcome studies can go a long way.

STRATEGIES FOR CONCEPT DELIVERY

In developing marketing strategy, you should focus on delivering these messages:

- Knowledge
- Accessability
- Quality

PHYSICIAN PROFILE

Physician name: _____

Does the physician have more than one office location: Yes or No

Primary Address: _____

Phone: _____

Fax: _____

Office staff names: Manager: _____

                                   Nurse: _____

Optimal time to visit: _____

Appointments or vendor slots: _____

MEDICAL BIO:

Board Certified/Eligible—Specialty: _____

School: _____ Residency: _____

On staff at these hospitals:

Medical director positions at:

Partner in practice/medical director At:

_____

Types of patients seen in practice:

_____

Approximate Payor mix of practice:

Medicare: _____ % Commercial/Indemnity: _____%

Medicaid: _____ % Workers comp: _____ %

Managed care: HMO: _____ % PPO: _____ %

Refers patients to (circle): Type/Diagnoses: Provider of choice

SNU   Y/N

Opt geropsych   Y/N

Inpt rehab   Y/N

Opt rehab   Y/N

Home health   Y/N

Inpt geropsych   Y/N

Cardiac rehab   Y/N

Personal info:

Married: Y/N   Spouse's name: _____

Children: _____

              _____

              _____

              _____

Hobbies: _____

Comments: _____

             _____

             _____

Additional Information:

_____

_____

Every aspect of the marketing effort, every promotional tool or event ties into these concepts. In working with physicians, many organizations get the physicians involved in the programs through such avenues as medical director positions, participation in different community marketing events, case studies on their patients, and reports back to the physician for the patients office chart. All of these in some fashion reinforce the concepts. Information and samples of tools can be found throughout this book, with discussions of them within Chapter 20, "The Marketer's Toolbox."

SUMMARY

The physician-marketing process is the same, no matter which product within the continuum is being promoted. The keys to success are the following:

- Develop a product and entire continuum knowledge to be most helpful to the referral source.
- Set goals and maintain a rotation schedule based on strategy.
- Don't personalize any outcomes that are less than expected.

15

CHAPTER

External Territory Planning: Building the Bridge to a Consistent Marketplace

Paula Lodes

Healthcare agencies must strategically identify and capture their markets to survive fierce competition. Yet planning to succeed in these fierce markets takes skill, persistence, time, effort, and expertise. All of these are important components not always available, or at best, difficult to enlist. In the past, hospitals have relied heavily on internal referral development to feed patients directly into their respective specialty product lines. Inpatient services are fed directly to various parts of a hospital by admissions to acute care units of the hospital. This practice is enhanced by the recruitment of physicians both general and specialized to the hospital staff. However, as the trend of shrinking acute hospital admissions continues, agencies must focus on external territorial planning strategies as a source of referrals.

In this chapter, we will explain in detail the process of developing an external road map that will lead referrals to your facility. Building relationships needed to establish the framework of success takes enormous time and energy and can be a source of extreme frustration before a sense of success is achieved. Creating the framework of successful referral development can be compared to the building of a bridge used to link cities together. It seems to take months and possibily even years to complete. But once it is complete, the traffic flows effortlessly across its span. The goal of this chapter is to organize and illustrate the components necessary to create the framework of a successful networking referral system.

KNOWING YOUR TERRITORY

In healthcare the product line is usually a service to the client, not the traditional product you can see and touch. Even though marketing and sales approaches to selling a simple product are similar in some ways to selling a service, in other respects they are quite different. Marketing and selling a product line of a service-related industry is far more complex. Product lines for service-related industries are complex because of the nature of the product. They must rely heavily on people to deliver the product. The service product must be monitored closely by management to deliver quality outcomes that will attract new customers. Arriving at the end result of a quality service product delivered by a friendly, pleasant, competent, and respected employee is in itself an art—the beauty of the service-related industry.

A key in delivering an exceptional sales response to your product is an in-depth understanding of the market your product serves. External territorial planning must begin with an in-depth examination of the service territory. Obtain a simple, enlarged map of the geographic area and plot your territory. It is appropriate to maintain a broad scope. Examine the area for geographic landmarks such as mountain ranges, rivers, plains, and such. It may seem irrelevant to study these factors. However, the target population may not choose to or be able to travel over extreme barriers to receive your service. If this is the case, no tactical strategy will allow results to be achieved. The density of population will establish the distance your product will travel. If the market is a densely populated area, results will be best in a smaller geographic area. If the population is more rural, then a larger territory will be necessary to compensate. In years past, healthcare agencies, out of respect for their neighboring competition, limited the geographic range in which they marketed for customers. However, the practice of limiting territories does not seem to be valid in today's competitive marketplace. Your competitor is in your own backyard!

Notice the flow of traffic within the territory itself. Where are the major highways? What cities and towns do they flow in and out of? Is the area served by a major highway or is it more local? In a service-related product industry, these factors are extremely important. People will not seek care in an area where travel is difficult. The most common customer of healthcare is the senior citizen; thus, accessibility is essential. Quickly identify factors that will enhance the flow of traffic, such as schools, universities, industry, and retail shopping centers. This exercise will prove not only helpful in determining your territory, but it will identify potential markets for advertising your product. And now for the difficult task: mark your competition. Everyone has competition. Unfortunately, some of us experience more than others. Competition is a double-edged sword. On one side it keeps our product lean and mean, trustworthy and efficient. On the other, it robs us of referrals and potential customers.

KNOWING YOUR COMPETITION

Competitive analysis is a vital key to your success. In addition to marking the location of the competition on the territorial map, get to know the source well. If you are new to the area, simply visiting on-site will prove very helpful. However, if you are acquainted with the competition, you will already have developed an opinion, good or bad, regarding their services. A helpful hint to prevent you from a predetermined opinion is to have a friend visit the facility for you. Elicit their responses and impressions. The same can be true for your facility. Have the friend anonymously visit your facility. How do you compare? This practice will prove valuable in identifying and addressing internal problems.

It is helpful to know the competition's history. When did they begin offering the service? Do they hold special recognition in the form of accreditations? Do they offer a specialty service? Are their employees satisfied in the workplace? Do they experience high staff turnover rates? The answers to these questions will identify potential strategies for development in the catchment area. As it relates to the development of external territories, it is essential to know the pattern of client flow. Where do the clients enter the system and what is their pathway of progression? The most efficient method of obtaining valuable answers to these questions is to travel into the market, interviewing and asking questions. This in turn will offer a better understanding of the market territory and serve as an initial contact with your potential referral sources. Strategically plan to conduct interviews to determine not only your market share but the competitor's share as well. Developing an understanding of the client's perceptions and the referring agent's impressions and insight into the competitor's outcomes will prove extremely helpful as planning commences.

KNOWING YOUR PROSPECTIVE CLIENTELE

Census-tracking information is readily available to determine where the target populations are located. The product service must be matched to a particular age category where the majority of clients will be obtained. For instance, if your service best serves the aging population, then search for the territorial areas where the seniors are located. More precise information is also available to help match product to client or vice versa. Determine what information will be helpful to draw a clear picture of the territory. Use the information to develop strategies that will focus marketing efforts. Remember, most tactical plans have price limitations. Spend your dollars wisely. Shop to find the most highly saturated age-specific target population areas.

With today's enhanced database systems, seemingly overwhelming amounts of information can be retrieved from your market area. The healthcare industry is no exception. Today the implementation of various healthcare services are based on intensive research known as demand studies. Very simply, what is the demand for the service being offered? Healthcare-related industries are required to submit information to governing agencies serving the population. The majority of this information is available to the public if the information deals with government finance or reimbursement of Medicare dollars. There are also companies who will supply demand studies for a fee. Demand studies simply cross-reference census information with the current financial trends in a particular area. The information can be taken one step further to include disease processes. The Medicare DRG classification system can be cross-referenced with the amount of money spent on a particular disease in a specified area. This information is helpful to determine expected trends. DRG-based demand studies are somewhat unlikely to deviate from existing trends unless the area in question experiences an outbreak of an unusual disease. Likewise, strategic plans must consider this information to project potential business.

Investigate within the territory to determine the current referral trends. Is the service you are promoting already available? Where are people being referred to for that service? The best method for achieving reliable answers to these questions is to conduct your own survey. When the issue of survey is initially addressed, you might be inclined to develop a written questionnaire and distribute it to the involved parties. But would this yield the valuable information needed to make appropriate conclusions about the market? Probably not. Besides, the return rate for questionnaires is not significant enough to support a valuable decision. Most significantly, written questionnaires do not evaluate or test for the presence of politics between referring facilities. One-to-one interviews with referral sources is the best method to retrieve valuable information. The interview also provides the opportunity to meet potential referral sources and to begin the development of a relationship. One of the most important skills a marketing person demonstrates is not his or her ability to sell the product but the ability to determine the needs of the client and what resource will best suit this need. The successful marketer asks more questions seeking knowledge and explanation than just informing his audience of the product he has to sell. There will be a special time reserved for a product infomercial. Referral sources, especially in healthcare arenas, are interested in quality, service, and dependability. If the service they are currently using provides these three factors successfully, then a different approach will need to be formulated.

Referral sources vary depending on the service product line. Identify early all the potential referral sources and be creative in the listing. Be careful not to exclude any potential referral sources. Determine the level of the referral source as primary, secondary, or tertiary. Primary referral sources are those who will refer to the program on a regular basis. These are the bread-and-butter sources for the product line. A great deal of time and effort will be invested into keeping these sources satisfied with the service. Secondary sources refer to the program on occasion. They are considered to be a good source of referral but may not typically see a consistent number of clients for whom the program is designed. The tertiary marketplace generally consists of the public as a whole. The situation usually drives the tertiary market level of consumer, not the volume. For example, a person may only be generally aware of the service offered by a healthcare agency until a close friend or relative is affected by a situation.

To remain focused on the market, list the key players, their locations, and their level of required marketing effort. Develop action plans quarterly that will encompass each of these referral sources and their respective level of marketing effort. Action-plan development will be addressed later in this chapter.

KNOWING YOUR PRODUCT

An in-depth understanding of the product line is necessary both at local and national levels. Staying abreast of trends in the appropriate fields of expertise is essential to provide a top-notch, respected product or service. The American public has come to expect quality and rightfully so. A job worth doing is worth doing well. A product ultimately can be enhanced by building a successful team. As mentioned earlier, you can only be as good as the product you are selling. The art of managing people to commit to quality and friendly service is often difficult to develop, but it can be done. The service-related industry must rely on people to deliver an all-encompassing product reliability. The most successfully marketed target areas are the results of careful planning from the ground floor up. They start with a well-trained, efficient team who work well together in mutual respect. The effective team will not only take on the product as their mission but will also become active in the marketing of that product. It is important to involve every member of the team in all aspects of a strategic marketing plan.

Build trust and reliability into the program, especially in the area of outcomes. No one goes into a store to purchase an expensive item expecting it to be inoperative within a short period of time. The same holds true for service-related product lines. The outcomes must stand on their own. Programs are available to evaluate client-centered outcomes and service satisfaction. Referral sources need to be kept informed of these outcomes so they can take ownership in the program. If they feel they have an integral part of the end result, they will continue to support the program by referring clients. As you build trust in the program itself, you must build trust with your potential referral sources. It is essential to do what you say you will do.

CASE STUDY

My mission was to enhance referral development for a newly opened rehabilitation unit. The territory consisted of a fairly evenly proportioned age census. Competition was one-sided. And of course, as you may have guessed, the referrals were not coming to my particular unit. The competitor hospital's rehabilitation center was, to say the least, a gorgeous facility. The territory had several small rural hospitals within its midst, most of which had affiliations with the competition. This was icing on the cake. Their administrative team had done a great job of securing the referrals by forming affiliations with the smaller rural hospitals. However, after months of interviewing and making initial contacts with the referral sources, I discovered that employees at the small rural hospitals felt threatened by this entity. The smaller hospitals' staffs felt the competitor's rehab unit was not offering a quality product to their patients. After all, rural areas are known to protect their neighbors. The final blow in this scenario was the "stealing" of the rural hospital's customers as they were discharged from the rehab unit. Instead of the competitor hospital referring clients to the smaller rural base, they were referred directly to the competitor's home health agency and subsequent product lines. This angered the referring hospitals. With knowledge of the situation and politics in mind, strategies were implemented to build a mutually respectful relationship with the rural referral sources. First and foremost, our hospital chose to build one of the finest rehab teams available. With the sincere dedication to service in mind, and a one-to-one relationship established between referral source and rehab team, we asked for our first referral and received it. Subsequent successes led to the establishment of a solid referral system built on mutual trust and respect. Even though the rehab team was responsible for the patient for only the short time of the rehabilitative stay, we still respected the "home base" of that patient. We returned that patient to the referring hospital's services. And soon we found that other facilities in the area felt the same way. It was not long before the external territorial market was referring to the "underdog." Build lasting one-to-one referral source relationships that are based on mutual trust and respect as well as a strong passion to meet the needs of the referral source and its client. The results will prove outstanding.

FORMING A PLAN OF ACTION

Tailor the strategic plan to meet the needs of your referral source. Business action plans are important tools to help keep us focused on the job at hand. After careful analysis of the market is complete, begin with an overall plan to encompass an entire year. This will serve as your business development plan. It should consist of a historical view of the facility. Describe the internal workings of the facility and detail extensively the service you plan to market. Be sure to include any team-building exercises and objectives you have identified for your unit. Summarize these factors and specify strategic goals to be accomplished within a suggested time period. Include statistical data to support goals the unit has set. Develop a detailed timeline with the stated strategic action plans. Creativity should be at its best for this section of the business development plan. Be sure to combine local and national aware-ness campaigns into the plan. The plan must encompass all potential referral sources from the primary, secondary, and tertiary levels. It should not only identify the potential referral source but also the fre-quency with which that source will be visited. Create a sense of direc-tion to the business plan by including a "position statement" for the marketing tactical plan. This statement should be brief and precise, stating the direction the product line will take over the next year. Even though the team might have developed several objectives they wish to accomplish, select three or four specific attainable goals and elaborate with specific interventions. The appendix of the document should in-clude all statistical data such as demand studies, census and age popu-lation figures, financials, referral and admission data, conversion rates, and at least a twelve-month trend of unit performance.

Seasonal action plans are developed with a shorter time period in mind. They account for events specific to the area and time of year. These are usually developed and implemented quarterly. Likewise, the seasonal plan should include a schedule of potential contacts and the frequency the contact will be visited, as well as scheduled events mar-keted to the secondary and tertiary levels. Again, the team should be included in all activities. Special events are enjoyable to create because they involve the clients, customers, their families, referral sources, and the staff. The more involved the parties become in the program, the more a sense of ownership will begin to grow, leading to growth and expansion. If expansion is present, then more clients will be able to participate and subsequently benefit from the program's valuable re-wards. Ultimately, the seasonal plan will coincide with the overall mar-keting business plan as if two images were overlaid to appear as one.

Schedule special events throughout the year to promote the vari-ous aspects of your well-developed program. These should also target the different levels of contacts. Primary-level contact events should address the problems or issues facing this level of referral source. For example, primary-level sources are usually caseworkers, discharge planners, or social workers who help strategically guide clients through the healthcare system. After careful assessment from this level, design an educational offering that addresses their identified needs. Obtain a speaker for the event and tailor the event to their needs. You will find the response to be far greater than your expectations.

Here is an example of a special event for primary-level contacts. Discharge planners and social workers experience a great deal of stress associated with their profession. With this thought in mind, a three-hour seminar was planned in their honor. First of all, the seminar was scheduled for only three hours, with lunch included. Why? Because of the nature of the personalities of most discharge planners and social work personnel, they feel accountable for their clients. They do not like to be away from this responsibility for long periods of time. The event, thus, was scheduled to begin in midmorning, allowing for the social service workers to check in and settle any pressing issues. The lecture began at 10:30 A.M. As an added incentive, the session included "guided imagery," a technique used by therapists to reduce stress levels. The participants learned various methods to help control and reduce their stress levels. A special catered lunch was provided, complete with door prizes, all targeted toward making the participants feel special. After a short break, they were presented with a success story involving a registered nurse who reduces his stress level by marathon running. To conclude the seminar, we provided the participants with a relaxing chair massage and sent the case managers home limp as wet noodles, with significantly reduced stress levels. The purpose, of course, is not to get tangled in the particulars of the special event, but instead to focus on the perceived needs of the participant and the target audience you are serving. By the way, referral sources were committed to sending their patients to our quality program as a result of their perception that this event was helpful. Routinely offer events such as this to your territory—at least semiannually.

Tertiary sources, primarily involving the public, are interested in the types of services offered, education regarding the service, and perhaps a demonstration. Most healthcare organizations participate in health fairs. Health fairs are a good method for informing the public of the services you provide. They allow you to distribute helpful information. And, they provide one-to-one contact between your personnel and the general public. However, health fairs can be expensive if they are not pushed to another level of information. You must be creative if you plan to receive any business from a typical health fair event. Get specific in the setup. Offer specific health fairs on such topics as arthritis, cardiac disease, stroke, support groups, or orthopedic problems. Make the disease-specific health fair a screening event. If you plan to market several product lines at one event, do so by having the event be interactive. In other words, have the target market participate some way in your program. Minilectures, demonstrations, and screening events are all examples of an interactive approach. Response to your event will increase if well-known physicians or healthcare professionals are involved in the presentation. Create the physical layout so that registration is required for participation. This gives you the information needed to form future mailing lists and to follow-up with a thank-you note for participating.

Church and civic organizations always welcome noted speakers to their meetings. They are a great vehicle for keeping your public informed of the service you offer. If your service contains a team of healthcare professionals, then you can schedule several different sessions on their respective areas of expertise. Remember to supply a token for participants to take home with them to remind them of your service or how to access the referral process.

MAINTAINING RELATIONSHIPS WITH SOURCES

Frequent contact with potential referral sources is one of the most important ways to develop successful external referrals. The one-to-one referral relationship is essential to the development and retention of a proven market. Scheduling quality time with the potential referral source regularly will demonstrate accessibility to the service, as well as prove sincerity. Address scheduling from two perspectives. One perspective is monthly, the other weekly. Begin each month with a review of the past month's activity. Determine the source of recent referrals and those of the past few months. Look for the consistent and inconsistent referral pathways to your unit. From this information, determine a rotating schedule based on a month. More consistently referring sources will probably need to be visited weekly, whereas less frequent referring sources could probably be addressed every two weeks. Most marketing and referral development professionals plan to be in the territory four days per week.

After a monthly plan has been established, break the calendar down to a week at a time. With today's computer capabilities, blank calendars can be personally created and lend themselves to an appearance of excellent organization. Superimpose the monthly calendar onto the weekly schedule. The monthly level should provide only the skeleton of the areas to be covered. The weekly schedule should contain the specific contacts. For example, if you plan to work in a particular area that contains all three levels of contacts, then merely list the area on the monthly calendar but list the specific contacts on your weekly schedule. Make your weekly schedule full of potential contacts. As you find most frequently, not everyone will be readily available to see you when it is convenient to your schedule. To ensure your schedule remains efficient, list as many potential contacts on your weekly schedule as possible. If one is not available to see you, then simply progress to the next on your list. Additionally, make your weekly schedules conducive to the territory. In other words, schedule contacts in a geographically close area to prevent unnecessary travel.

Identify rotating schedules early after initial contacts. Complete interviews and study past referral records carefully to guarantee you are focused on a particular goal in a specific geographic location. Time and experience in the territory are necessary to develop a complete rotating schedule. After approximately six to nine months of experience with a particular market, not only will the players in the various levels surface but the territories themselves will identify their own rotating schedules. If you can picture the solar system and the rotation of the various planets around the sun, then add the rotation of each planet around its own axis, you will grasp the concept of rotating schedules within rotating schedules. Just avoid becoming dizzy!

It takes time to develop one-to-one contacts, referral sources, and referrals especially if the market previously had not been developed. Added pressure is always felt when administrators are expecting results. Most administrators are not aware of the enormous amount of time, energy, and sometimes pure luck that go into the development of territorial markets. They merely see the end result of massive amounts of energy; the flow of referrals. Frustration is unavoidable. Time always ticks at the same pace regardless of the speed your feet are traveling.

What do you do with a potential referral source that never refers? This is always one source of immense frustration within every territory. Regardless of the time and effort you have spent establishing one-to-one working relationships and making sure the sources have been thoroughly introduced to your product, some don't refer a patient. Continue the normally scheduled contacts as you had planned, and when the time is appropriate, address the problem in a direct manner. Simply ask why. Most sources will tell you if higher politics are involved or if they are uncomfortable with the referral. Regardless of the reason, you at least know why. Now you can proceed with an approach or a solution. If the potential referral source is uncomfortable with the program itself, ask for a trial patient, then prove the outcomes. When hospital politics are involved, the process of receiving a trial client becomes tricky. It may require a phone call or an initial meeting between the powers that be at a higher level. Use perseverance to arrange a meeting between the parties, which can open the gates of referrals. Nevertheless, continue with the contact for a predetermined period of time. If the trend continues and you have found no apparent reason for the reluctance on their part to refer, then shift the source to a less frequently visited level and concentrate your efforts on more productive turf.

Primary referral sources are usually busy people working several different cases at one time. Any assistance you can offer them will help secure your overall rating with them. On numerous occasions, client evaluations have revealed results that are quite the opposite of what the case manager or family would like them to have revealed. This creates problems and frustration. The family and case manager were expecting a smooth transfer to your facility when, in fact, the patient does not meet criteria or would not be best served by your program. Whatever the reason, take the process further to assist both family and case manager. Do not leave the case manager with, "I'm sorry but Mr. Smith does not meet medicare criteria for admission. Call me when you get another referral." In reality, you probably would not address the referral source in such an abrupt manner, but in telling them the patient does not meet criteria and dropping the process at that point, haven't you done the exact same thing? Take the time to find a solution for that patient. Again, this proves to the referral source that you are sincere in your effort to put the client first.

Tracking the results of your marketing effort is essential. It not only proves your worth but provides you with helpful information that will improve the overall business plan. Enormous amounts of information can be retrieved with only a minimal amount of forethought and planning. Establish a method of tracking early in your efforts. At the close of one year, closely examine the results and search for patterns within your system. Share the information with the program team and see if they interpret the information as you have. Seek their input and suggestions for possible new avenues. Also, use the results to strengthen your value to the team and the overall program. The benefits are as numerous as you allow them to be. Often, the tracking system will need to be altered and enhanced as it grows with your market. Make the system work to your advantage.

CONCLUSION

This chapter has intensely focused on establishing and developing an external territorial marketplace. It is no easy ballgame to play. It requires skill, time, persistence, effort, insight, and patience to build a successful and consistent market. Begin with a plan—a comprehensive, realistic, obtainable plan. Discover the territory and the players. Search to find the underlying pathways that are dominating the current flow of clients. Work to establish a program of intense quality and reliable outcomes. Rally the team to help you tackle the obstacles you will experience along the way. Be there to witness the client and his family as they are victorious over the challenges of their lives. Promote the successes to ensure more.

16 CHAPTER

Marketing Assisted Living Services and Using Videos

With the aging of the population, assisted living facilities are rapidly proliferating. In a niche sandwiched between independent living facilities and nursing facilities, they appropriately fill the gap for those who either need assistance daily or who choose because of anxiety about their health issues to be in a facility that offers stronger support. Even this niche has subsegments. Some facilities offer basic care services while others offer add-on services at incremental fees and can provide much more extensive care.

Promotion of these services can be divided into two areas: external promotion (i.e., to the public and referral sources) and internal promotion of the facility (to families, visitors, volunteers, etc.) External promotion is a constant challenge because of the lower conversion rates of inquiries to leases, many may inquire or tour but not move in.

At any given time those making inquiries may not progress to admissions for various reasons, including three major ones.

The first is long lead times. The decision to move from one's home to a facility is not made hastily unless it is primarily driven by acute illness or one in which there is little hope of returning home. If the decision to move is made, many family members—and thus many conversations—may be involved. There may be the sale of a home, which may take six months to a year. The individual's health status may also change during this time.

A second reason that an inquiry may not lead to a lease is a misunderstanding about care levels that are provided or needed. This can be viewed as a question of how much help one really needs. This can be a difficult choice, especially if perceptions of capabilities are not consistent or if an individual's state of health is changing. It is also worth noting that individuals may be more capable and coherent at different times of day, and this can skew perceptions of the actual level of care needed. Because of this and other reasons, some inquiries regarding assisted living are directed toward nursing facilities. The third reason is the tenuous state of the frail senior's health. An acute episode may occur at anytime, thus altering the planned lease.

TARGET MARKETS

Hospital-Based Social Work or Discharge-Planning Professionals

Hospital-based groups, such as discharge-planning professionals, are traditionally reached by one-to-one education contacts. In many areas, and especially in metropolitan markets, these people have been so overwhelmed by marketers that they now refuse to visit with even those who are in the hospital assessing individuals. Needless to say, more creativity is indicated. Clever marketers now use the mail for delivery of newsletters, monthly calendars, and photos and newsclippings of events. Others, realizing that everyone has to eat, offer functions and "gourmet" breaks to secure time with these very important referral influencers. As you read through this book, there are many suggestions on working with this and all of our target markets.

Physicians and Their Office Staffs

Few physicians make house calls at assisted living facilities. Instead they rely on families and the facilities' transportation services to get patients to them. This is more economical given their daily schedules, but offers less routine interaction with physicians on the part of facility staff and marketers. Again, one-to-one calls on the physician or their office staffs can bridge this gap. As healthcare marketers have become more aggressive, however, they often find themselves waiting their turn on vendor day for increasingly brief visits. Many now recommend focusing efforts on the office staffs who interact with families, and who often provide them with a more informal referral information system. Some facilities deliver cards with photos of their residents (the physician's patients) in activities or out and about. (A resident must have signed a photo consent form, of course.) Sometimes the residents deliver the cards themselves during their regularly scheduled visits. This group often has established strong relationships with physicians and their office staffs.

The Public at Large

Open a newspaper almost any Sunday and most likely you will see a number of advertisements for assisted living facilities. It is imperative to establish a level of name recognition so that when people need the service they have a facility recognized as a provider.

As stated earlier, keep in mind that the decision-making process in this transition from home to an assisted living facility can be protracted, or a rapid one after acute illness. Given the nuances of the process, keeping your facility at the front of people's minds can drive site selection once the need is indicated.

There are also a number of persons who, by their involvement with facilities, influence referrals. These persons are frequent visitors and volunteers—guest artists, performers, or support group leaders. These individuals are generally involved with more than one facility and acquainted with residents and families at those facilities. These guests are in a unique position to promote one's facility from the inside out. Church groups often perform or clergy members conduct services. These same individuals, respected within the community, relate what they see and experience in facilities.

Travel Agents

For respite care, many assisted living and long term facilities market to travel agents. The rationale for this target market is that when families are interested in vacations, the travel agents can offer solutions to their concerns (such as a family member who needs care daily) and thus facilitate a respite that the caregiving family so desperately needs.

(Keep in mind that all other referral sources can also refer to respite care.) The respite stays may result in future residents.

INTERNAL MARKETING

It is also important to market internally. You can pour money into advertising, but the facility must show well daily, seasonally, and for special events.

On tours across the United States, we have seen many facilities with an internal marketing focus. Some touches are very effective, present well, are inexpensive, and are easily implemented. Many facilities include coffee or tea service in the lobby, as well as complimentary newspapers.

The ambiance of any facility can be enhanced by music. One facility we toured has classical music softly playing on the overhead speaker system. In addition, two stereos are kept on rolling stands to bring to activity areas or to the several dining areas. We were told that many of the residents seem especially to enjoy music from the forties; planners try to keep a variety of that music available in addition to the many entertainers who visit the facility.

Dining is a special emphasis for most facilities. Baby boomers who may have established expectations based on past paradigms are likely to be, at the least, pleasantly surprised and more likely shocked by the gastronomic offerings. Facilities are including extensive menus in their packets and touting "chefs hired from the restaurant industry," along with food service directors who are graduates of prestigious culinary schools. The fresh foods and from-scratch cooking may be better quality than that found in many families' kitchens that are frozen-food and microwave dependent. Do not expect to see paper, plastic, or mismatched place settings. These dining rooms often feature linens and fresh floral arrangements. One facility offered special monthly theme nights, with the management serving residents and guests, and also quarterly family nights. The quarterly megaevents feature a theme, associated cuisine, extensive decorations, and guest performers. For example, "Fiesta Night" included two chef-manned buffet stations, a menu to rival a restaurant, a mariachi band, a beer and frozen-margarita bar, and fantastic decorations. There were wooden cacti and candles on the tables (accompanied by chips and salsa), five-foot-tall cacti in the corners, Mexican vases, flowers, hats, and serapes strategically placed to enhance the atmosphere. The staff all dressed in fiesta garb to complete the theme.

Activities have changed, too. While the perennial bingo remains a favorite, we are now seeing much more extensive offerings to meet the desires of this new, more-demanding generation of residents. There are both more and a better variety of activities offered, with an increase in such offerings as community trips. These residents are alert and alive, relishing the freedom of participating in activities. Games may include card and board games, including bridge and many others, while sports may include exercise, bowling, or putting practice right inside the facility as a warm-up for the golf trips. These seniors are moving. It is likely that if you tour a facility, they will not only have the activities calendar for the month posted but will also include a copy in the inquiry packet. Many persons will decide on a facility based on the quality of the food and the activities if all other issues (location, cleanliness, appearance, etc.) are considered equal.

FACILITY PROMOTIONAL VEHICLES—VIDEOS

Considering the resources dedicated to the inside of the facility and the accoutrements, you might think that promotional materials would be minimal because the facilities can speak for themselves. But this is not true. These facilities need to be full, and as a result, the promotional materials are often even more expensive for this product. They are likely to be glitzier in their appearance. Full color and multiple promotional pieces in the inquiry packet appear to be the norm, not the exception.

We also have noticed a number of videos within the promotional effort. Consider, as we mentioned earlier within this chapter, that residential decisions may be made by multiple people and by those who may have paradigms regarding eldercare. Videos are one way to demonstrate clearly the new reality of senior care in assisted living. They are also helpful in our mobile society for family members who may be living out of the area.

We have included the scripts for three videos for one facility. The first script was developed to respond to inquiries. The focus facility presents very well, but in reviewing inquiries during our analysis, it was found to have a low conversion rate (inquiries converted to admits) when no tour was conducted. We will review several other contributing factors in Chapter 19 within the section on competitive analysis and inquiry assessment. Within this organization there are different levels of care, from assisted living through skilled care. The facility offers the residents the opportunity to "age in place," move from one level of care to another when necessary. The executive director plans to mail the video to those persons who request information and thereby hopes to impact the conversion rate.

As you read through the video script, look for the food and the activities. As we have stressed in this chapter, these are two paramount areas for this product. Throughout the video the facility reputation is stressed, both through the use of references (television and magazine) and the support of the residents and families. The facility presented well, but it was also important to stress points that the viewer cannot see. The concept here was that of "picturing yourself or someone you love" at the facility, with shutter sounds and photographic terms interspersed. This concept also was chosen specifically to control costs with less intricate editing requirements.

Video 1: Facility Inquiry Video

Concept: Picture yourself here

> **Voiceover:** *(First and last name),* **executive director (holding a magazine)**
> Hello, and thank you for your inquiry regarding *(facility name).* I'm *(first and last name)* and I would like to take just a few minutes of your time to help you picture our facility. We are very proud of the facility, and we should be. In 1994, *(name of TV station's)* investigative reporter, *(name of reporter),* reported that *(facility name)* was "operated like a facility should be." In their June 1996 article, *(name of article),* the *(name of magazine)* expert recognized *(facility name)* as the "place where he would put a relative of his own."
> **[shutter sound; external shot of building]**
> *(Facility name)* is located just off *(street name)* between the intersections of *(street name)* and *(street name).* The facility is set off of the thoroughfare, away from the hustle and bustle, yet conveniently located for visitors and families.
> **[shutter sound; external shot of building with name visible]**
> As you approach the building from the south, you will see the two-story brick building with our name, *(facility name),* in

white letters on the side. We have designated parking in the
front for the convenience of families and visitors. Visitors are
welcome anytime, but we do ask that you respect other residents. Remember, this is their home.

[shutter sound, shots of lobby, front parlor, and office area]
You will notice that we are very different. Our facility is small,
elegant, and homelike. We offer public areas such as parlors
and sitting areas so that our residents may entertain guests
as they would in their own homes. Our administrative suite is
just off the front reception area, and we have an open-door
policy for families and residents. Even on weekends, a member of our management staff is available to focus on your
needs. Just stop by the office. (*Magazine name*) commended
us in their (*issue number*) issue for our consistent management. I have been the administrator here for four years and
the owners of (*facility name*) are (*city*) residents themselves.
In fact, they also rotate weekends and holidays as the managers on-site. They care about their homes and their residents, just as all of our employees do.

[shutter sound, event pictures in the front lobby]
(*Facility name*) can accomodate 150; however, because so
many residents select private accommodations, we are usually full with only 95 residents. This means we have a very
cozy and personalized environment, and our staff develops
caring relationships with their residents. Our residents are at
varying levels of independence from those who are almost independent to those who depend on our staff of professionals
for every aspect of their care.

[shutter sound, transition to conference room]
This room is available for the use of residents and their
guests, private dining, or small parties. It can be a cozy atmosphere for a quiet conversation or a family celebration. It is
equipped with a VCR for screening those home movies of special family events.

[shutter sound, shot of first-floor nurses' station]
The nurse's station is located adjacent to the elevator on the
second floor. Our nurses are on duty twenty-four hours a day,
seven days a week. Many of our more independent residents
have chosen (*facility name*) because we do have nurses on-
site for quick response. Our more independent residents live

on the first floor, with the residents who need more intensive care on the second floor. All our doors and elevators are accessible by code for the security of all residents.

[shutter sound, shot of smiling employee helping resident in the hall]

(*facility name*) is proud to deliver special care in an elegant atmosphere, but it is our employees who make it so special. All candidates face an extensive interview process with the management team, and I personally interview all prospective final candidates for positions. Many people apply for jobs with our established and reputable facility, but we pride ourselves on choosing the right candidates and making the best possible decisions. (*Magazine name*) in its (*issue number*) issue recognized our employees as the most helpful, with a low turnover rate.

[shutter sound, shot of the kitchen, vegetables being chopped]

Our dining room is the setting for exceptional dining comparable to many (*city name*) restaurants. Our meals feature fresh fruits and vegetables and "scratch" cooking, a pleasant surprise for our resident's guests. Our food service director is a graduate of the Cordon Bleu School of Cooking in London, and our staff has both long-term and restaurant experience.

[shutter sound, shot of the dining room]

Guests may join residents for daily meals for a nominal charge, and menus are posted weekly. Additionally, we feature monthly theme nights and quarterly family nights. You probably noticed the picture board in the front lobby with our most recent events.

[shutter sound, transition, courtyard shot, include doghouse]

Our large courtyard is a tranquil oasis, with sitting areas and a water garden surrounded by lush vegetation. (*facility name*) landscapers ensure that the area is in bloom all year round. It is a picture-perfect setting for relaxing or joining in activities, and is completely wheelchair accessible. The water garden was a gift from a family of a former resident. She loved the courtyard and now her gift makes it even more special. Residents may smoke out here if they choose. Lucy, the (*facility name*) mascot, has her official place of residence out here, and often visits our residents.

[shutter sound, shot of first living area]
We have several types of personal living areas available. Our residents arrange and decorate their living spaces as they wish; we have asked two of our residents to share a peek at their areas. Residents may choose to bring their own furniture or just use ours and bring personal items from home. It is important for residents to be comfortable and happy, and we encourage them to make this their home. Our belief is that our residents don't live in our facility—we work in their home.

[shutter sound, shot of second living area]
Each living area has a response system that provides immediate communication. It is not simply a call-light system but a two-way speaker system. Our residents' living areas are cleaned by our housekeeping staff, and the maintenance staff handles preventative maintenance and any necessary adjustments. Each room has individual climate control for maximum personal comfort. We can provide full laundry service in addition to linens at no extra charge for your convenience.

[shutter sound, shot of loading the van to go out]
Our activities department at (*facility name*) conducts events throughout each day on both floors of the facility for all residents. Each day's events are posted by the elevator, and may include games, spiritual sessions, in-room movies and visits, or guest entertainers. Every month we sponsor a birthday party and a welcome event for new residents. The "out to lunch" bunch meets once a week, and excursions are planned to local sites of interest. Our van service is wheelchair equipped so that all residents may join in the fun.

[shutter sound, transition to name of executive director in front of framed article in his office]
I hope you have enjoyed this brief look at (*facility name*). We are a small facility offering personal attention to our residents. Our residents usually come to us through word of mouth, and we would be happy to provide names of family members and residents who act as our references. Our setting is not right for everyone. But if you can picture yourself or someone you love at the (*facility name*), please phone me or my assistant administrator, (*first name last name*) at (*phone number*) or just stop by and see us at (*address*), right here in (*city*).

The film was hosted by the facility's executive director and constantly referenced points of quality and reputation. This executive director realized before the marketing competitive assessment and inquiry study was conducted that the facility's biggest referral source was word of mouth from families, residents, and individuals who were acquainted with the facility. He wanted to market to this all-important group. His final decision was to construct a video that could be shot in-house with his own video camera, featuring the management team. The focus of the video was ostensibly to introduce the facility's management team and services. But the video is also a strong marketing piece both to reinforce the difficult choice made and encourage confidence so that the viewers will refer others.

The second script was developed for the families of newly admitted residents to acquaint them with the management team and the features of the facility. As you read, you will note that the video has three purposes. The first is to educate, the second to manage or set expectations, and the third is to market the facility. The video markets the facility by sharing information that families should be aware of—for example, that the executive director personally interviews all final candidates and conducts quality assurance rounds. As you review this video, you can discern the marketing focus but will no doubt benefit from insight into facility operations, as a family member would. Each department manager was filmed in his or her office. Picture yourself in their shoes.

Video 2: Orientation and Marketing Video for New Residents and Their Families

[Department—Activities]

Hello, my name is (first name last name) and I am the activities director here at (facility name). Our residents enjoy participating in a variety of activities just as you do. We offer games such as bingo, Wheel of Fortune, and card tournaments. Our sports here include putting practice and bowling. We keep residents apprised of current events with special taped presentations, as well as through the local newspapers. Here at (facility name), we offer spiritual programs in addition to Sunday services, bible study, and readings from publications. Each month we offer special theme nights and a birthday party. Throughout the month we feature many guest entertainers. Some of our residents choose to participate in outings and excursions to local points of interest. We have a van equipped for wheelchairs and bench seats so that everyone may enjoy our outings. It is important that we know what activities our residents enjoy, so please share preferences or your knowledge of your loved one's favorite pastimes. We encourage residents to participate and enjoy socialization. Some individuals prefer more solitary pursuits, so we offer our book cart, in-room movies, and visits. We have something for everyone! Monthly activity calendars are included in our newsletter, and invitations are mailed for special events. Guests are always welcome, and events are announced over the speaker system. We in activities look forward to having you join us.

[Department—Human Resources and Staffing]

Hello and welcome to (*facility name*). I am (*first name last name*), the human resource and staffing coordinator. My role here includes interviews and reference checks to be certain that our employees are very special. Many people apply for work here at (facility name), but we try to select only the very best, the kind of people that we all would want to take care of our family members. In addition to my human resources role, I also coordinate the staffing for the facility to ensure that we have adequate numbers of staff, scheduled and present on every shift to deliver the type of care that we demand and our families expect. Thank you for choosing (*facility name*). I will be working behind the scenes to ensure we are staffed with the right people to deliver care to our residents.

[Department—Medical Records and Central Supply]

Hello, my name is (first name last name) and my responsibilities here at (facility name) include central supply and medical records. You see, before a resident even comes to (facility name), we make certain that we have any special supplies on hand that they may require when they arrive. Our goal is to provide a seamless care transition. A new resident may need a special mattress, incontinence products, or dressings. Throughout the stay they may require nutritional supplements or other special care products, such as a wheelchair cushion.

We serve as a resource for families to order items, as well as providing for residents' daily care needs. I'll be here working behind the scenes to ensure that your loved ones have all of the supplies that they need as part of our quality care.

[Department—Assistant Administrator]

Hello and welcome to (*facility name*). My name is (*first name last name*) and I am the assistant administrator at (*facility name*). My primary role is to assist residents and their families with any concerns or issues they may have. We help families through their move in transition and on an ongoing basis. Tours and inquiries are another major area of focus for me. Because of the care provided here and thanks to the very special employees who deliver this care, practically all of our referrals are by word of mouth. That makes us very proud, and it is always a pleasure for me to handle an inquiry or tour when someone is interested in placing a loved one here.

I also supervise the housekeeping, laundry, and maintenance departments, and with those departments will work closely to ensure that you or your family member are comfortable at all times. If you have any questions or if I can help you in any way, please phone me or stop by the office.

[Department—Maintenance]

Hello, my name is (*first name last name*) and I am the maintenance supervisor here at the facility. You may not realize just how much is involved in maintaining a quality facility. On a day-to-day basis we address items in need of attention and conduct preventative maintenance. Daily quality-assurance rounds identify areas of focus, and we can start on them immediately. By keeping daily tabs on our facility we can be certain that everything is in tip-top shape for the benefit of our employees and residents. If I can provide any assistance in a resident's living area, please phone or stop by the front office and notify a member of the management staff.

[Department—Front Office]

Hello, my name is (*first name last name*) and I am the office manager here at (*facility name*). As part of my responsibilities, I manage the front office, which includes communication with families, answering the phone, arranging guest meals and reservations for special events, and handling all of the billing for the facility. I work closely with (*first name last name*) in Central Supply and Medical Records to make certain that every bill is accurate. If you have any questions about your account, or if I can help you in any way, please phone or stop by the front office.

[Department—Nursing]

Hello, I am (*first name last name*) and I am the director of nursing for (*facility name*). Ultimately I am responsible for all the nursing care provided for our residents. I work closely with the staffing coordinator, (*first name last name*), and the executive director, (*first name last name*), to make certain that our care is first rate—the kind that everyone would want for their parents or grandparents. Quality assurance is a big part of what I do—checking the quality of our care and our documentation, and making certain that we comply with state and federal regulations. I work with the staffing coordinator to make sure that everyone here has education in specific areas so that they can be the best they can possibly be at caring for residents. If you would like to discuss our nursing care, I will be happy to help you. I have an office on the second floor near the nurses' station, or you may just ask the front office personnel to page me.

[Department—Executive Director]

My name is (*first name last name*) and I am the executive director here at (*facility name*). While I am ultimately responsible for the operation of (*facility name*), my duties vary from day to day. I work with families, taking inquiries regarding their needs and services here at (*facility name*), and I conduct tours so that people considering staying here can really see the facility and meet the employees who deliver the fine care here. One of the areas I enjoy the most is interviewing every employee who joins us at (*facility name*). I feel strongly that it takes special people to deliver care in our special setting, and by intensively screening and interviewing prospective employees we can ensure that we find the very best team members. I also lead quality assurance rounds with the management team. We visit with all residents and their aides to determine the conditions of residents and the physical plant so that we are truly apprised of care and can maintain the standards that we have set. We conduct these rounds on all shifts, and many are unannounced rounds. If you have any questions or concerns please don't hesitate to phone me or stop by my office. Even on weekends, a member of the management team or the owners of (*facility name*) are available to meet with you.

[Department—Food Services]

Hello, my name is (*first name last name*) and I am the director of food services at (*facility name*). Here at (*facility name*) we serve approximately 350 meals every day. Our challenge is to serve nutritious, delicious meals, on time and at the correct temperature. We have a dietary consultant who works with us to plan caloric and nutritional intake. Our food will probably not be what you are expecting. I am a graduate of the Cordon Bleu School in London, and we recruit chefs from restaurant settings and serve fine quality meals such as what you would order when you go out. Residents here enjoy fresh fruits and vegetables, and our meals are made from scratch. We offer two entree choices for meals, and can provide substitutes if a resident declines the choices. We even keep snacks so that residents can snack at different times of the day, just as they would at home. From early morning to 6 P.M. you may get coffee and tea from the kitchen, and there are vending machines in the rear hall behind the kitchen. After the kitchen closes, visit the nurses station for coffee or tea.

You are welcome to join us for meals. Just call or stop by the office and they will notify us. There is only a nominal charge for guest meals, and you may pay either at the front office or we can charge your account. We look forward to seeing you.

As you noticed in this video, there was significant repetition of the facility name and cross-referencing between managers of other department managers' names and titles in order to build recognition. The video reinforces the quality of the facility without constantly stating, "Aren't we great?" There is no doubt that a family member or new resident will be better familiarized with the facility and that they have been very effectively marketed to. At this point the Executive Director, who knew the value and associated costs of scriptwriting, decided to modify the family and resident video for use in new-employee orientation. Employees are a significant marketing vehicle in both conveying our messages to residents, families, and visitors, as well as to these same groups in other facilities as they change positions. (Refer to Chapter 11, "Internal Marketing Opportunities to Strengthen the Continuum of Care.")

Review the following third script, comparing it to the previous script. The executive director of the facility was well aware that video production has an estimated cost of approximately $1,500 per minute. He felt that he had invested time and resources into the project, and with a minimal additional investment, the script could do triple duty! This is a very economical use of dollars. This version was filmed in the conference room used for orientation sessions, and the department heads were thus excused from routine appearance at every orientation. Given the unexpected challenges that arise daily in the healthcare setting, all of the managers expressed a sigh of relief about the filming instead of being negative regarding the project.

Video 3: Modified Version for New Employees (Internal Marketing)

[Department—Activities]
Hello. My name is (*first name last name*) and I am the activities director at (*facility name*). Perhaps you are wondering just what our department does and how you may interact with us in the course of your job. Our residents enjoy participating in a wide variety of activities just as you do. Every day our list of activities is posted and we announce activities prior to their start time. In addition, we will apprise you and the residents of activities during quality assurance rounds in the morning. Please help us to encourage and help residents to activities. We will be depending on you to know which of your residents can be encouraged to participate and to make a difference in their lives by getting them involved in socialization and leisure activities. From time to time we may even ask you to lead an activity, and we hope you will enjoy doing so.
[Department—Human Resources and Staffing]
Hello, and welcome to (*facility name*). I am (*first name last name*), the human resource and staffing coordinator. I am an LVN by background and have probably already spent time

with you during our interview process. My role here includes interviews and reference checks to be certain that our employees are very special and that we only hire the best. Many people apply for work here at (*facility name*), but we only select those who we feel are the best. In fact, that is why you are here. We think you are the best. In addition to my role in human resources, I also coordinate the staffing for the facility. Staffing levels are important to us and our residents, so if you have an emergency that prevents you from working your shift or causes you to be late, please call us as soon as possible. Our residents are our priority and we must cover your shift, so please do call us. The protocol for calling in is: Please phone the nursing station or the office two hours prior to your shift so that we may fill your shift with a co-worker who would like to work. Vacation requests are submitted to me. I also coordinate ordering uniforms. I look forward to working with you and am glad that you've chosen us here at (*facility name*).

[Department—Central Supply and Medical Records]

Hello, my name is (*first name last name*) and my responsibilities here at (*facility name*) include central supply and medical records. As part of medical records, I maintain active charts, periodically thinning them and maintaining old chart information to adhere to regulations. We also keep every daily assignment sheet for staff and all of the inactive charts. In central supply I interact with all facility personnel, ordering supplies that we all need to carry out our duties and keep (*facility name*) running smoothly. We ask here that you sign out supplies. It is important that you know that we stock supplies on the floor once a week. If something is needed, tell the front office so I can replenish the supply. I hope you like working at (*facility name*) as much as I do.

[Department—Assistant Administrator]

Hello and welcome to the (*facility name*). My name is (*first name last name*) and I am the assistant administrator. My primary role is to assist residents and their families with any concerns or issues they may have. Tours and inquiries are another major area of focus for me. Because of the care provided here, by employees just like you, practically 100 percent of our referrals are word of mouth. That makes us very proud and it is always a pleasure for me to handle an inquiry or tour when someone is interested in placing a loved one here. Tours are where each and every one of you can participate. When you see a tour being conducted, please act just as you always do—smiling and greeting all our residents and families. Sometimes I will stop and introduce employees to families touring because I am so proud of the facility and staff. Don't be surprised if you are participating in my next tour! In my position I handle the day-to-day facility financial duties such as balancing the facility accounts, reviewing invoices, and issuing employee loans. My office is in the administrative suite if you need to stop by. If you notice anything that needs our attention, please call or bring a note to me so that we can keep (*facility name*) in tip-top shape! I look forward to working with you.

[Department—Maintenance]

Hello, my name is (*first name last name*) and I am the maintenance supervisor at (*facility name*). You may not realize just how much is involved in maintaining a facility like (*facility name*). On a day-to-day basis we address items in need of attention and conduct preventative maintenance. Daily quality assurance rounds identify issues that we can begin on immediately. These may be small issues, like hooking up a new resident's television, or something that needs quick repair. By keeping daily tabs on our facility, we can be certain that everything is in shape for the benefit of our employees and residents. If you see something that I need to work on, please notify (*first name last name*), the assistant administrator in the front office.

[Department—Nursing]

Hello, I am (*first name last name*) and I am the director of nursing for (*facility name*). Ultimately, I am responsible for all of the nursing care provided for our residents and work closely the staffing coordinator, (*first name last name*), and the executive director, (*first name last name*), to make certain that our care is the kind that you would want for your parents or grandparents.

Quality assurance is a big part of what I do—checking the quality of our care as is reflected in our documentation to make certain that we comply with certain state and federal guidelines that apply to patient care in nursing facilities. If you are in the nursing department, the chain of command for issues is as follows: nurse's aide and medication aide, to charge nurse, to assistant director of nursing, to director of nursing. If you are in the nursing department and must call in sick for a shift, you should call the charge nurse on the unit at least two hours before your shift begins. A member of the nursing management is always on call so that we can quickly call one of your co-workers to cover a shift. We hope you enjoy working at (*facility name*) and look forward to having you join our patient-care team. We hope to have a long relationship with you in a work environment that you will enjoy.

[Department—Executive Director]

My name is (*first name last name*) and I am the executive director here at (*facility name*). While I am ultimately responsible for the operation of the facility, day to day my duties vary. I work with families, taking inquiries regarding their needs and services at (*facility name*) so people can see the facility and meet the employees, like you, who deliver our care here.

One of the areas I enjoy the most is interviewing every employee who joins us at (*facility name*). I feel strongly that it takes special people to deliver care in our special setting. By interviewing prospective employees we can ensure that we find the very best team members to join us, folks just like you. I lead daily quality assurance rounds with the management team. We visit with all residents and their aides to determine the conditions of residents and the building so that we are truly apprised of care and can maintain the high standards that we have set. If you ever have a problem or concern come talk to me—we can talk in confidence and take care of almost anything.

[Department—Food Services]

Hello my name is (*first name last name*) and I am the director of food service at (*facility name*). Here at the facility we serve approximately 350 meals per day. Our challenge is to serve nutritious, delicious meals on time at the right temperature. We have a dietary consultant who works closely with us to plan caloric and nutritional intake. If you have worked in other facilities, you will probably be pleasantly surprised by our meals here. Today, as a new employee, you will be our guest in the kitchen for a complimentary meal. As an employee you are welcome to eat here for a small fee, but the cafeteria is only open to employees for meals between the times of 11:15 and 11:30 A.M. and 12:15 to 1:30 P.M. for lunch and 5:30 to 6:30 P.M. for dinner. We are serving residents meals at other times and will serve employees on a different schedule. Be sure to bring your meal ticket to the cafeteria; no employee can be served without a ticket. Coffee and tea are available daily from 5 A.M. until 6 P.M. at no charge in the kitchen. It is important for all of our staff to know that we offer substitutes for residents if they do not care for either of our entrees. Snacks are available for residents in the refrigerators on the units, as well. Vending machines are located on the first floor near the activities department. We are glad you've chosen (*facility name*) and welcome you to our team. Stop by and join us at mealtime!

In this video again we see the repetition of names and titles for the new employee's benefit. The video emphasizes the fact that only the best are hired at the facility and reinforces their choice to apply and work at the facility. At this focus facility, the assistant administrator has a commitment to getting employees involved on tours and thus apprises them of tours and their potential involvement. The expectations for call-ins are identified and restated, even though they are part of other areas of the orientation day. The orientation video has a number of advantages and can be produced in conjunction with a family/new resident video economically.

COMPETITIVE AND INTERNAL ASSESSMENT

While all managers are presumably proud of their facilities, the managers who have a marketing orientation also will be intensely interested in their competition. Members of the administrative community are often well acquainted with each other and do visit competitive buildings. In addition, many managers employ a friend, family member, or consultant to conduct competitive assessments.

Obviously, the competitive assessment indicates how the focus facility compares to the competition, and more important, how the focus facility can position itself to more effectively compete. The assessment for this facility is included in Chapter 19, "Competitive and Process Assessments."

CONCLUSION

Marketing the assisted living facility, especially if there is an extensive service diversification, is a multifaceted undertaking involving the entire staff. Use the techniques discussed in this chapter to inspire you, whatever your setting may be. Remember, referrals can come from almost any source, but we must infuse a sense of pride and confidence in our employees and in those who entrust their care and the care of their loved ones to us. The focus facility in this chapter does indeed get its referrals from word of mouth and has emphasized the provision of quality care for years. However, as more competitors with newer physical plants enter the market areas, even the best must work harder.

CHAPTER

Marketing the Skilled Care Unit

William E. Brady

So, you've just landed that great job you've been trying to get forever. You've been named marketing representative for the skilled care unit. It is time to prove to everyone that you can make an impact. Now that you have a basic understanding of what it takes to qualify a patient for admission to your skilled unit, what do you think should be done next? Where will these patients come from and how will you let them know that your unit can meet their needs? How are you going to determine when you will have beds available? Better yet, how can you keep yourself focused on the task of attracting patients, educating referral sources, and assessing the needs of these same referral sources? The referral sources will be consistent whether the unit is hospital based or within a freestanding facility.

REFERRAL SOURCES

The desirable patients are going to come from a variety of hospital-based sources—hospital based because they have to meet the Medicare skilled qualifier to be accepted. The logical place to start is within your hospital, or if the unit is freestanding, at the local acute care and specialty hospitals. Concentrate on those facilities that are within twenty miles of your facility. List all of these facilities and note if they have any specialty units such as acute rehab, geropsychiatric, or even their own skilled care facility. Make a note of whether they have a large physician following in orthopedics, neurology, and cardiology. Do they have other specialty programs such as a cancer center? All of these programs will be opportunities to market and educate. Get a list of the physicians on staff at each hospital. This is usually readily available from the physician-relations department. Target all physicians who will be seeing the type of patients you are going to be providing services for. Each of the potential referral sources listed below will need your attention:

- Physicians
- Discharge planners
- Social workers
- Seniors' groups such as AARP and Sunday school groups
- Senior citizen centers and ministerial alliances, and other sources

Physicians

Physician referral sources can be divided into two classes according to their clinical specialty: decision makers and influencers. Decision makers are usually primary care physicians such as family practitioners, internists, and general practitioners. These physicians have a history with the patient and family and will play a strong role in determining their postacute care. Do not overlook the office nurse or the office manager. These people can become your best friends when it comes to the ability to interact with physicians. On the initial office visit meet or at least get the names of the physician's nurse and office manager. Follow-up visits are much easier if you are dealing with someone on a first-name basis. A colleague of mine has developed the technique of placing his appointment calendar on the desk open to the appropriate month. He then asks the receptionist or whoever is manning the desk if a certain date is good to see the doctor and, if not, if he can set another date. He gets an appointment about 70 percent of the time. Another marketing method is to arrange to bring in lunch for the staff. I have done this with good results in the past. I do not even ask if the physician is going to be available. I want to make friends with his or her staff. I do try to determine when the doctor eats lunch and schedule my staff visit at that time. Always be sure you have provided additional lunches, in case of unusual circumstances. On one occasion the physician I wanted to see had a colleague visiting him who I also wanted to meet. Both physicians joined us for lunch and I was able to communicate to them how our program could benefit their patients. On another occasion the physician's wife and oldest son were visiting. We had an excellent meeting and I learned a lot about this physician. During the course of your visit look for the following:

- What type patients does this doctor see the most?
- What hospital(s) is he or she affiliated with?
- Is the physician part of a larger group?
- Are they approved providers on managed care plans your organization deals with?
- What can you and your program do to help them and their patients?

This information should become the basis for your needs analysis or an answer to this question: "What does my program offer to these physicians that will help them give their patients better care?"

Influencers for the most part are specialists such as orthopedic surgeons, vascular surgeons, and neurologists. These physicians may have less control over where a patient is discharged for postacute care, but they often recommend providers. Given that they do not always have direct control over the patient's discharge destination, how do we get them involved? One good way is to get them involved as a consulting rehab medical director. In this role they will be a key player in helping your team develop the best patient care possible. They can also play an important role in your marketing efforts by interacting with other physicians in the area. Another good strategy is the formation of a physicians advisory board. Putting a small group of physician influencers together for the purpose of evaluating your program and suggesting ways it can change for the betterment of the patients and the community is an excellent way to give them ownership and to enhance your marketing efforts. There are other ways to get these influencers on your side; we will address them later in the chapter. Remember, just because you may never see a direct referral from these physicians, they still play an important role in your success.

Discharge Planners

Without a doubt, discharge planners are probably the single most in-fluential group you will deal with in your marketing effort. It is esti-mated that in some hospitals, discharge planners play a pivotal role in up to 50 percent of the placement of patients in the postacute care con-tinuum. Who are these people and what makes them tick? Medicare was created in 1962 in an attempt to provide all of the healthcare cov-erage Americans needed. It did not take long for people to realize that Medicare, as it was created, could not fulfill this role without some cost constraints. This realization lead to the creation of the diagnostic re-lated group, or DRG, system to control Medicare costs.

Who has the responsibility to try to see that patients do not ex-ceed their DRGs? The discharge planner. These individuals usually find themselves caught between the physicians, who do not feel their patients are ready to leave the hospital, and the utilization manage-ment or review group, who are monitoring the appropriateness and cost of the length of stay. They need you to respond quickly to their requests for an assessment and to give them an answer as quickly as possible. What they really want to do is to turn this patient or that pa-tient's discharge plan over to you.

Is this marketing? You better believe it is. You want to prove to them that not only is your program the best suited to meet their pa-tient's needs but that you understand their problems and can help solve them. How do we do this? In much the same way we approached our physicians. Arrange in-services at their convenience to explain your program and at the same time find out what kind of system is in place. In some hospitals discharge planners have responsibility for an entire floor, such as surgery or medicine. In one large facility I am fa-miliar with, discharge planners are assigned to specific physicians. Whatever the system is, be aware of how it works.

The next step in this process is the most important one in deal-ing with discharge planners. You must implement a system that allows you to respond to their requests faster than your competition and to have an answer for them without undue delays. I know of one contract management company on an inpatient unit that did not respond to discharge planners' calls for twenty-four to forty-eight hours within their own facility. They lost that contract. This can clearly impact cen-sus. Discharge planners must be educated about the admissions process. Facilitating an admission to a hospital-based subacute or skilled care unit can be different from arranging admission to an SCU that is part of a long-term care facility. It is important that they understand the unit's admissions process. This does not mean they are not going to call you at 5 P.M. Friday with a referral and that you are not going to do everything you can to accommodate them. Educating them will, hopefully, help everyone to plan ahead.

Another good marketing tool you can use with discharge planners is to invite them to participate in in-services that your facility or program has scheduled. This will give them a clearer picture of how you are preparing your staff to meet their needs and the needs of the patient. Asking them to be a member of the advisory board is another example of how you can get them to participate in your program. Their input is important in helping your program stay abreast of the hospital's or community's needs; that is how you should approach them.

Social Workers

Social workers have a good bit of influence on family members and the decisions about a patient's aftercare. Many hospitals use social workers as discharge planners because of their ability to help people make decisions in difficult situations. Acute inpatient rehab units employ social workers to lead the discharge process. Inpatient SCU units are required to have a social services assessment done within forty-eight hours of admission. These people should not be ignored in our marketing approach. They need to be as aware of what your program can offer as a physician or discharge planner. Since there will be fewer of them in the facility you are marketing to, take the time to find out what their role in the discharge process is. Provide them with printed material that they can use appropriately with family members and patients. Include them in in-services for discharge planners, or, better yet, conduct an in-service just for them. Do the same kind of needs analysis you would do for the discharge planners and compare them. There will be differences to be aware of. Offer to take them on a tour through your facility and have them join you for lunch in the facility dining room with the patients. Your efforts here are centered on them developing a sense of comfort with what you can offer and relaying that sense of comfort to their patients and families.

Seniors' Groups

Seniors groups such as AARP and senior Sunday school classes are another potential source of referrals. These are people who are well and do not particularly want to think about a hospital stay, but are likely to know someone who is ill. Approach them from the standpoint of community service and education. Ask for permission to speak to their group on the programs you can offer should there ever be a need for your services. Take along your nursing or therapy staff members and present a program to inservice them including exercises for back pain or stroke prevention and awareness. Provide them with printed material that they can keep for future reference. You may not be able to track specific referrals to these groups in the future, but their influence can be helpful.

Senior Citizen Centers, Ministerial Alliances, and Other Sources

Every community has a senior center and a ministerial alliance, although it may not have a formal title. These are influencers in the truest sense of the word. The senior center is a place where many of your discharged patients meet for activities. They are always willing to allow you to do educational meetings for the benefit of their members. They also will be happy to come and talk to your patients about what they can offer them after discharge. Many times the senior center operates the special needs transportation system, especially in smaller communities. Think of ways you can tie them into your program. One way would be to arrange for them to pick up some of your patients who are able to go on community outings for lunch or to spend time in an activity. Ask them to help you with an event that you are planning to draw attention to a healthcare issue. I once requested that the local senior center provide transportation for a wheelchair scavenger hunt our hospital unit sponsored during National Rehab Week. We took a group of local business leaders and politicians, put them in wheelchairs, and transported them to a local mall where they had to obtain items without leaving the wheelchairs. It was a great success.

The ministerial alliance can be a formal or informal monthly gathering to discuss all sorts of topics. Ask them if you can come to a meeting and provide them with information on your program. Involve one of them on the advisory board. The chaplain at one of your referral hospitals should be able to direct you to the alliance.

Other potential referral sources are home health agencies and medical equipment suppliers. Home health agencies are in a unique position to help you build your census, especially when you are just starting to market your program. They are called on to assess patients in the hospital who have to be discharged but who often are not really ready to go home, even with home health. Home health agencies can refer these patients to you, but are also competing for referrals. You will want to develop a relationship with several agencies so you can ensure that all your market is covered. Medical equipment suppliers are another source of market information. They are involved in the discharge process and can provide you with information about program changes you might not be aware of. Remember, it is very important that you recognize shifts in your market before they occur so you can plan your strategy.

DEVELOPING A MARKETING PLAN

Now that you have identified the people and organizations that you are going to market your SCU to, you need to develop a focused plan. This marketing plan has to have specific, achievable, measurable goals, and a time frame for reaching these goals. You can use many types of marketing plans, and you have to be comfortable with the one that you choose. I have seen beautiful plans that were fifty pages long with graphs and charts and bound in a leather binder that were worthless. Once they were written they were left on a shelf to gather dust. A marketing plan's value is in being used. It needs to change with the market and it should be anticipatory or proactive. The correct marketing plan can put you on the road to success. The marketing plan I like contains the following elements:

- Summary of the program being marketed, including any past performance history
- SWOT (strengths, weaknesses, opportunities, and threats) analysis of the program (internal)
- SWOT analysis of the competition (external)
- Action plan

Program Summary

I like to start with the program summary to focus on what I have to offer. Performance history, if available, can help you look at past trends that may have affected the program. You can identify seasonal swings in census or identify problems with referral sources. Except in cases of units that have just opened, there should be records to review that identify referring physicians and facilities, diagnoses most often seen, and which physicians no longer refer. The summary should also include facts about your facility. If your facility is located in an acute care hospital that has just completed a cancer center, it should be noted in your summary. If your facility is in a long-term care setting that just added a therapy gym, note it. The summary should also provide information on facilities in your immediate area. This information is available from the American Hospital Association but can also be obtained from the public relations department at the various facilities. Call the local chamber of commerce for the latest demographic information. All of this is important in the beginning to build your marketing plan.

SWOT Analysis (Internal)

The next step is a SWOT analysis of your own facility or unit. Look at what you have to offer the community (strengths). This should include special programs you offer such as wound care or pain management. Do you have a full-time therapy staff? Who are your medical directors, and are they well known in the community? Do you accept HMO/PPO plans that are currently in your community? What is the ambiance in your facility like? Is your facility new or old? Are you hospital based, part of a large national chain (premier reputation, ability to attract the best employees) or are you a mom-and-pop shop (lots of hands-on care, part of the family)? In short, what do you have to offer? It does not have to be different to be a strength.

Now you need to look at weaknesses. You might say that your facility does not have any weaknesses. But if I do my job well, I am going to find my competitor's weaknesses and turn them into my opportunities. Be realistic. Your competitors know if you have weaknesses and they are trying to use that to their advantage. Use it to your advantage instead. By understanding a perceived weakness, you can put a positive spin on it while marketing before your competition turns it into an opportunity for them. For instance, you have just heard that your competition is emphasizing that your facility does not have a van for community reentry. This comes up when you are visiting a discharge planner.

What do you do? One way to combat this is to tell the discharge planner that your unit uses transportation locally, either through the senior center or department of aging, for community reentry. This is better for the patient because the new van at ABC facility will not be available for patients to use once they are discharged. You are helping patients learn to use what is available in the community. You should note the weaknesses and attempt to enhance services whenever possible.

From weaknesses we go to opportunities. Take advantage of those market shifts. Opportunities come in all shapes and sizes. They can be good or bad. Analyze them carefully. Having a van to use for community reentry probably seems like a good opportunity. If there are alternative methods that you can use that enhance your program as well, look at them too. Does the gain justify the cost? An outpatient therapy program in a long-term care facility may sound like an opportunity, but not if you do not have the therapists you need to run it. Accepting respiratory patients to your SCU can be an excellent opportunity. In a hospital-based setting it is fairly easy to do, but in a long-term care setting the start-up may not be worth it. Do not promise a program or service that you cannot deliver. One facility I am familiar with began to promote respiratory rehabilitation months before they could be ready. Soon they were getting respiratory referrals, including vents, that they could not service. The damage done to this facility's reputation was significant. It took a lot of hard work on the part of the marketing person to get back on the list with discharge planners. Be careful that your enthusiasm does not create problems. Finally, be aware of threats to our program. These threats are market changes and fluctuations. For instance, you have been told that DEF hospital is planning to open their own SCU. DEF is one of your primary referral sources, and any unit they open will adversely affect your unit's performance. The unit will open in approximately a year since you are in a certificate of need (CON) state. You want to assess the damage that could be done to you immediately by assuming the worst-case scenario. What is your potential loss in revenue if you get no more patients from them? What can you do to lessen this impact? Are some of your primary referring physicians affiliated with this hospital? What is their opinion of the hospital's move? Can they still be counted on to support your unit? These are questions you have to answer about any threat; you have to be ready to combat them. This illustrates the importance of a flexible, proactive marketing plan.

SWOT Analysis (External)

Now perform a SWOT analysis on all of the competitors. Any facility that has an SCU in your geographic area (remember we said twenty miles) should be included. Look for the same information. Why should someone refer patients to them? Do they have programs you do not? Do they have a strong physician base? Who is their medical director? What kind of programs do they offer? Do they have any weaknesses that you can turn into opportunities? For instance, do they use PRN therapy while you have a full-time therapy staff? Do they have an RN running their unit? Can they take respiratory patients?

What are your opportunities? Now you have changed the nature of your questions. What do they not do that you can turn into opportunities for yourself. Once again, be honest. What threats do they present to your program? How can you overcome these threats? Do not be afraid to change the marketing plan.

Action Plan

This is where Clark Kent comes out of the phone booth and smites the forces of evil. So Clark, what can you do now? Now review the program summary and the internal and external SWOT analysis to set some goals. Remember that the goals must be specific, achievable and measurable within an established time frame. A three-month period works best, with continuous review monthly. Set achievable goals for yourself as well. It is very frustrating to feel that nothing has been accomplished because goals are unattainable. Do not set yourself up to fail.

The following is a marketing plan for the hypothetical facility.

Sample Marketing Plan

Summary

XYZ Care Center is a 150-bed long-term care facility with thirty licensed Medicare beds. The facility was built in 1995 and is located in Jonesville, a town of 80,000. There are three acute care hospitals located within twenty miles of the facility, one that has a twelve-bed skilled care unit. The latest census figures for this area indicate that 27 percent of the population is in the 65-and-older age bracket. The facility had a small (twelve beds) SCU until it was renovated in 1996. Average daily census (ADC) for the SCU was nine patients and the average length of stay was thirty-two days. The facility enjoys a fine reputation with the local medical staff.

SWOT Analysis (Internal)
Strengths

- Subacute unit
- Therapy gym with complete activities of daily living (ADL) kitchen and bathroom
- Physiatrist as rehab medical director
- Respiratory therapy twenty-four hours a day
- RN Medicare coordinator on staff

Weaknesses

- Weighty admission process
- Perceived as a nursing home and not a rehab center
- Staff turnover is high

Opportunity

- Streamline admission process
- Change perception of community by offering rehab education

Threats

- DEF hospital to expand skilled unit

SWOT Analysis (External): One major external competitor
Strengths

- Excellent community reputation
- Strong physician following

Weaknesses

- Older physical plant
- Several physicians retiring
- Staff turnover is high

Opportunities

- Market newer state-of-the-art facility
- Physiatrist to take stronger role in marketing

Threats

- Expanding SNF

Action Plan

Goal	Action	Time	Result
Change community perception of facility	Develop new collaterals	11/96	At printer
Streamline admissions process	Shorten process by combining forms	12/96	Ongoing

This is a very simple marketing plan that combines all the elements we have discussed. Develop your own plan and use it. Failing to plan is planning to fail.

MARKETING COLLATERALS

Marketing collaterals are used to enhance your program and to educate your consumers. A simple brochure that tells the story of your program is effective. Develop your collaterals so they can be used with referral sources and patients and families alike. It is more cost-effective and a better use of your resources.

CONCLUSION

Be flexible as you develop plans. If the plan is not working, change it. Do not let your ego lead you to failure. Review the plan often; it is the key to your success. Look at it daily and make notes on it. It is a tool, just like a hammer or a saw. Use it like one.

18

CHAPTER

Managed Care and Marketing the Continuum

Edward M. White

Managed care organizations design and evaluate their networks of healthcare providers on the bases of quality, reputation, accessibility, and price. Consider a four-legged stool with each of the legs representing these factors. Each of the legs is equally spaced, and equally long and each is required for the stool (the managed care network) to stand alone. For this stool to support the care delivered within the network, each of the legs must be sturdy. If any of these legs is thinner, shorter, or weaker, the managed care network will not support the covered lives and will therefore topple.

In the beginning of managed care development and until the 1980s, these networks were fairly small. During the 1970s and 1980s, employers saw their healthcare benefits costs rising. These decades were marked with annual increases of as much as 25 percent. As the cost of delivering healthcare rose, employers increasingly sought out managed care plans that offered relief from the spiraling costs.

Early efforts at managed care included benefit provisions for pre-certification of treatment and second surgical opinions. These programs were aimed at reducing medically unnecessary treatment. Today, the second surgical opinion program is virtually gone, since costly surgery does not seem to be so unnecessarily prescribed.

However, precertification is still required by most insurance programs and managed care plans because it assists in identifying the most appropriate treatment setting.

Today's managed care programs are typically recognized as including preferred provider organization (PPO), point-of-service (POS), and health maintenance organization (HMO) plans. PPOs are generally thought of as the least-restrictive managed care plans; HMOs are generally considered the most restrictive. Each of these offer features for controlling the cost of healthcare and ensuring delivery within the most appropriate treatment setting for the best possible outcome.

Typically, PPOs offer the covered individual an incentive to select a network provider through benefit incentives, where in-network benefits are 10 percent to 20 percent higher than out-of-network benefits. PPOs must have large, broad-based networks of providers for the patient to have a reasonably large number of choices in the healthcare treatment. Of the managed care plans, PPOs offer the largest degree of choice to the patient. Because of their structure, PPOs access standards are relatively high—acceptable access standards with X miles, where X is smaller than for other managed care plans. However, with a large number of providers, the tolerance for price is slightly wider.

At the other end of the managed care spectrum are HMOs. HMO plans typically offer the strongest incentive for a patient to select a network provider—100 percent in network and no coverage out of network. HMO networks are typically smaller than PPO networks, since the covered individuals must select an in-network provider. In addition, HMOs typically require covered individuals to see their primary care physician (PCP) first. PCPs direct the care of the individual either through their own practice or by appropriate referral to a specialist. These PCP gatekeepers are encouraged through incentives to provide treatment themselves for all appropriate conditions. HMO networks are typically smaller with greater tolerance for access; however, the tolerance for price is less.

POS plans are in between PPOs and HMOs. POS plans are termed such because the benefit is determined at the point of service. They typically have a gatekeeper primary care physician requirement, a strong incentive for the patient to select a network provider, some out-of-network benefits, and medium-sized networks of healthcare providers. Covered individuals seek initial treatment from their PCP, who treats or refers to a network specialist. In this instance the patients receive in-network benefits and the employer/insurer enjoys network pricing. When covered individuals self-refer to a specialist, they receive out-of-network benefits. If the specialist is out of the network, the employer/insurer must accept out-of-network pricing. Under this plan, a covered individual may be referred out of the network by the PCP, with in-network benefits received by the covered individual but out-of-network pricing experienced by the employer/insurer. POS plans are competitive with HMOs in controlling healthcare costs and still offer a choice to the patient.

Today, managed care plans cover a significant portion of the commercial population. As a result, healthcare providers who have chosen not to participate in managed care networks are seeing more of their patients directed away from their practices than ever before. While trends indicate that healthcare providers who have participated in managed care plans early benefit most from managed care plans, more providers are interested in and seeking membership in managed care networks.

In many areas of the United States, managed care plans may have closed panels of network providers. In such instances, providers outside of these networks will not have access to as many potential patients. More patients now recognize if and when they have a choice in a health care provider, and they are more likely to seek treatment from a specific practitioner if they are offered incentives.

In order to appeal to the managed care network, it is important for healthcare providers to understand a managed care organization's business environment. Since managed care plans develop and maintain their networks on the bases of quality, reputation, accessibility, and price, a healthcare provider should market its continuum to managed care plans on these bases. Healthcare systems have greater appeal to many managed care plans than do individual healthcare providers.

QUALITY

The first leg of our managed care stool is quality. The quality of care delivered in a managed care organization depends on the quality of the healthcare providers in the organization. Managed care plans have long been attacked on the assumption that the quality of care delivered in the organization must be substandard. Managed care organizations "credential" their healthcare providers both prospectively and retrospectively to ensure high quality. Thus, to gain and maintain membership in a managed care organization, healthcare providers must continually demonstrate high quality of their services by objective means.

Independent quality assurance organizations are expanding today to meet the demand for independent quality ratings of healthcare providers. Many managed care organizations require accreditation by organizations including the Joint Commission for Accreditation of Healthcare Organizations, the National Council for Quality Awareness, the Health Care Financing Administration, the American Hospital Association, the American Medical Association, and the College of American Pathologists. Some of these organizations are government agencies; others are independent private agencies supported by members. Managed care organizations have reviewed their requirements for membership and rely on these agencies' reporting mechanisms to credential healthcare providers. Continuums of care are challenged to require and maintain records regarding the quality of its members.

Managed care organizations are interested in having healthcare systems in their networks. Healthcare systems offer several advantages to the managed care organization, including singularity of contact for a number of healthcare providers, peer pressure for maintenance of high quality standards, and ease of referral within the system. Increasingly, managed care organizations are seeking out these continuums.

Quality is also reflected in a healthcare provider's business practices. Many managed care organizations use information systems that facilitate profiling of healthcare providers. These profiles measure and rank a provider's clinical practices and business practices. For instance, a surgeon's profile may include a measurement of the appropriate use of assistant surgeons. Other quality measures in a provider's profile may include a measure of appropriate level of coding for the service provided to patients. Managed care organizations may track a provider's adherence to the terms of the managed care agreement and include that information in the profile. While these profiling systems are relatively new for managed care organizations and healthcare providers, they are mainly used to provide information that will allow the providers to improve their practices. In the future, these profiles may be used as a standard of membership in a managed care network. Quality is not limited to clinical measures.

Managed care plans encourage their members to seek care from a network provider by offering higher benefits for in-network care than for out-of-network care. This redirection of members may be viewed as vouching for the quality of the network providers. Thus, managed care organizations carefully prospectively and retrospectively review the credentials of network providers.

A healthcare system should give strong consideration to quality assurance and accreditation. As managed care organizations grow and direct their covered individuals to network healthcare providers, those providers maintain or increase their market share. Meanwhile, those providers not in managed care networks may be losing market share. Managed care organizations now require quality assurance and accreditation for membership in their networks. With so many healthcare systems and individual providers maintaining quality assurance and accreditation, managed care organizations can limit their networks with these requirements without losing reputation or access. Thus, organized healthcare systems that assure quality and maintain accreditation have an advantage and will likely benefit in the future.

REPUTATION

Reputation can be as important as objective attestations of high quality. If a managed care organization has a poor reputation, its popularity and therefore income will be reduced. A managed care organization's reputation is largely a result of the reputed quality of care delivered in the organization, and that reputation is derived from the reputation of the healthcare providers in the network.

CASE STUDY

A managed care organization entered into an agreement with a county hospital in a medium-sized Midwestern town. This county hospital is one of four hospitals in the local managed care network and one of seven hospitals in the area. The managed care organization views this hospital as appealing and as an asset to the network. It offers a wide range of services and is affiliated with a respected medical school. The physicians affiliated with this hospital are considered by the managed care organization to be on the cutting edge because of their affiliation status as instructors with a teaching hospital. However, many residents in the area discount the county hospital; they believe that because county hospitals have a strong responsibility to provide care to the indigent, the facilities and care offered through this facility must be sub-standard. While this perception is not accurate, the managed care organization's local network was not as marketable because of the reputation it gained by adding a county hospital to its network.

A number of health insurance agents and brokers were asked what factors, in order of priority, were important in the sale of group health insurance policies. Assuming all bids were close in price, having the "right" doctors was the number one factor. Thus, the reputation of the healthcare providers is important to the managed care organization.

Reputation can be a broad brush, with implications about such issues as quality, bedside manner, hours, and location. The well-run healthcare system will maintain high quality through rigorous independent standards review and will market itself as high quality. It often has the resources to feature good locations and the foresight to offer flexible service hours. It is likely to be well regarded, with documentation of good outcomes. Thus, good practices will beget good results, and those results will propagate a reputation that will attract managed care organizations. More covered individuals will be directed to the continuum of care system.

ACCESSIBILITY

As discussed earlier, managed care plans vary in regard to accessibility requirements. PPOs typically require better access than HMOs, with POS plans in between. For metropolitan areas, it would not be unreasonable for a PPO to have at least two primary care physicians within eight miles of every member. A healthcare system offering the continuum of care should offer accessibility for the population they are targeting.

Accessibility, too, has more than one meaning. Access is necessary for managed care networks to be marketable; groups are not interested in offering an incentive that cannot be easily achieved. Additionally, access is important to achieve treatment easily by high-quality, reputable network healthcare providers and thereby to realize the potential efficiency. Further, with competing managed care networks offering easy access to groups, access has become a requirement for the marketability of the managed care plans. Accessibility may not be just a measure of the distance to travel to a network provider, but also a measure of covered individuals' ability to use their healthcare benefits.

If the continuum of care system is interested in becoming a provider in a managed care organization, it should learn about such areas as the managed care organization's members, their market area, and the organization's accessibility standards. With this information, the continuum of care system will be able to measure itself against these standards and appeal to the managed care organization by demonstrating its fulfillment of these standards. The highest-quality, best-respected providers may not offer access for a managed care organization's members and therefore would be less attractive than a continuum of care with access.

PRICE

The last leg of the stool for managed care organizations is price. Managed care organizations are often a part of one or more health insurance companies. These companies are in the business of selling health insurance. Increasingly, these policies are managed care plans. Competition in the area of health insurance is fierce with the advent of numerous managed care organizations. Group health insurance is typically offered by an employer to its employees.

Employers are easily able to secure bids for their health insurance policy today because of the large number of insurers. This competition and a demand from the employers for more from the insurance carrier has pushed managed care organizations to ask for more from the healthcare providers in their networks. As insurance companies are preparing quotes on health insurance, they must project expected claims for the group. To best project claims, insurance carriers and managed care organizations must know what healthcare services will cost. Thus, while managed care organizations were willing previously to base agreements with healthcare providers on a discount-from-charges basis, they now require an agreement that specifies a specific dollar amount for a specific service. Additionally, managed care organizations may base their agreements with healthcare providers on a payment of a given amount regardless of the service provided, or payment per member per month (capitation). In any case, these agreements allow insurance carriers and managed care organizations to better project claims for a group of covered individuals. As they are better able to project claims, they have more confidence in aggressive pricing of their insurance policies. This should result in more sales and growth of the managed care organization.

Fixed pricing is important to insurance carriers and managed care organizations, as well as to healthcare providers. In preparing a bid or reviewing a rate schedule for a managed care organization, providers must determine the appropriate payment level. A healthcare system should determine how much new business the managed care organization can direct to its healthcare providers or how much of the system's existing business could be lost if the system were not a part of the managed care network. What is the benefit structure for the plans offered by the managed care organization? What amount of redirection will these benefit structures provide? How many competing health care systems/providers are going to be in the network and who are they? Do the terms of the agreement with the insurance carrier or managed care organization extend only to those benefit structures with redirection, or will the prices apply to nondirected (indemnity) covered individuals? Additionally, what is the long-term projection of membership for the managed care organization? Will it grow in the future? Many in the healthcare/insurance industry expect to see managed care plans with some choice (out-of-network benefits) for covered individuals to be the long-term winners. Most expect indemnity (non-managed care) plans to disappear in the near future. Managed care organizations with large membership or large potential whose plans have strong redirection obviously are interesting to healthcare systems and should be courted. This is the point at which effective use of the continuum services can have strong appeal in managing costs by treating patients in the most appropriate yet cost-effective setting.

Price is probably the one leg of the stool with elasticity; if all other factors (quality, reputation, and accessibility) are present, a managed care organization probably has some flexibility in its price agreements. A healthcare system offering a continuum of care that can be contracted through a single agreement or just a few agreements, that has high-quality care as attested by independent accreditation, that has a good reputation in the community, and that offers accessibility to potential and current targeted patients can probably negotiate better payment levels than an average group of healthcare providers. This level of elasticity in pricing varies depending upon the managed care organization and the type of managed care plans offered.

Managed care organizations develop their networks to sell more health insurance. The organizations must sell more policies to generate more revenue, and develop win-win relationships, as in Figure 18–1. To accomplish this, managed care networks must meet the needs of the policyholders. Policyholders are interested in lowering their healthcare costs. Healthcare costs can be lowered through directing covered individuals to network providers. Because this direction of covered individuals may differ from what they would otherwise select, these providers must be of the highest quality and be accessible. Alternatively, some covered individuals may choose to select a non-network provider for some or all of their healthcare treatment. In this instance, managed care plans must offer an out-of-network benefit. In consideration for this redirection of covered individuals to network healthcare providers, the managed care agreement requires participating healthcare providers to agree to accept a specific fee for specific services, where that fee is lower than the healthcare provider would charge otherwise. If these conditions cannot be met, all parties lose (Figure 18–2).

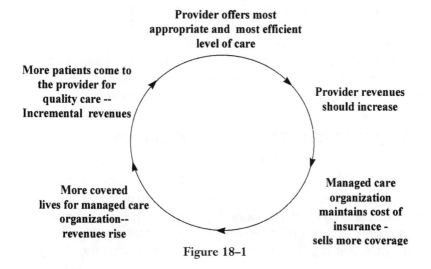

Win --- Win --- Win

Provider offers most appropriate and most efficient level of care

More patients come to the provider for quality care -- Incremental revenues

Provider revenues should increase

More covered lives for managed care organization-- revenues rise

Managed care organization maintains cost of insurance - sells more coverage

Figure 18–1

Lose --- Lose --- Lose

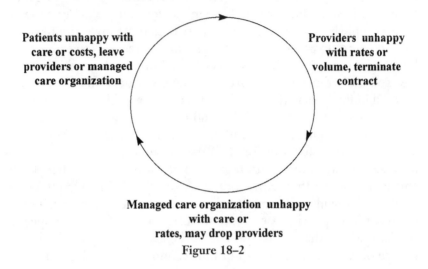

Patients unhappy with
care or costs, leave
providers or managed
care organization

Providers unhappy
with rates or
volume, terminate
contract

Managed care organization unhappy
with care or
rates, may drop providers

Figure 18–2

Healthcare systems should be interested in gaining and maintaining membership in managed care networks to increase or maintain market share. To gain and maintain membership in a managed care network, a healthcare system must get to know the managed care organization and market themselves to these organizations continuously. To market the healthcare system's services effectively, the system needs to know the managed care organization's requirements and business. Many health care systems create a position solely for managing the relationship with managed care organizations.

THE ORGANIZATION'S MANAGED CARE CHAMPION

An outward indication of the importance of a position is the reporting structure. If the position that manages the relationship with managed care organizations reports to the chief executive officer, it is an indication that managed care relationships are as important as operations and finance. The position responsible for maintaining the relationship with managed care organizations may be called director of managed care, managed care coordinator, or vice president of managed care. This responsibility may also be a part of business development, operations, or finance for the organization. Whatever the title, the person selected for this position must be knowledgeable of managed care both as an industry and within the market area of the healthcare system. This individual should locate and secure information regarding such issues as the type of managed care plans, the amount of redirection offered by each, the number of covered individuals for each plan, the reputation of each of the managed care plans, the standards for membership in each of the managed care networks, and the expected growth of each of the managed care plans.

The organization's representative should analyze this information and work with the management team for the healthcare system to select plans judiciously. Healthcare providers should not necessarily participate in all managed care networks. Once the managed care organizations are targeted by the healthcare system, the managed care representative should approach and make application to those managed care organizations. The marketing approach should demonstrate how the healthcare system will help the managed care organization meet its goals. The communication should not end when the contract is signed.

Once a healthcare system has gained an agreement with a managed care organization, it must continue to keep abreast of the changing needs of the organization so that it can look for opportunities to strengthen its relationship and to demonstrate how it continues to help the managed care organization meet its goals. With so many plans to participate in, a healthcare system offering the continuum of care must have a department that establishes and manages these relationships. This department may consist of one or more persons, depending on the needs of the healthcare system.

Many healthcare organizations have misconceptions about managed care. Some mistakenly believe that anyone can deal with managed care organizations. Without managed care expertise, the organization may have difficulty in its managed care relationships and may lose market share or miss opportunities to improve market share.

Managed care organizations and managed care plans cover a significant portion of the commercially insured population. Managed care plans already cover a growing portion of the Medicaid and Medicare population, and it appears that many uninsured lives will be covered by managed care plans in the future. Managed care plans direct their covered individuals to healthcare providers in their networks. Managed care networks do not typically include all healthcare providers. Therefore, providers in managed care networks are maintaining or increasing their market share while providers outside of networks are losing it.

SUMMARY

Managed care organizations design their networks on the bases of quality, reputation, accessibility, and price. Healthcare providers interested in joining or maintaining their membership in managed care networks should market themselves to the managed care organizations. By demonstrating the ability to meet the managed care organization's needs, healthcare providers are able to secure or maintain membership in a managed care network and therefore increase or at least maintain market share.

Health care systems offering the continuum of care have an advantage in appealing to managed care organizations. Continuums of care typically have greater ability to satisfy the managed care organization's quality, reputation, access, and prices standards, and have greater ability to demonstrate this need satisfaction continuously. This ability is typically facilitated through the designation of a department or an individual to focus on the managed care relationships for the continued success of the continuum.

19

CHAPTER

Competitive and Process Assessments

INTRODUCTION

Although we would all like to believe the *Field of Dreams* concept—If you build it, they will come—it is unfortunately not true. But as organizations chase their dreams of being full service, it is reasonable to assume that sooner or later there will be a program with difficulties (whether internal or external) that will seriously affect their ability to reach financial projections. Some situations will be confined to just one program or service component; some will be more systemic, based in the organizations' inquiry, referral and intake process, admissions process, or care-management routing system. In any event, it is paramount to success to identify problems in a timely fashion and to take steps to address them to improve performance. This is the most significant component of our business, and the one that we enjoy the most. Organizations are often successful in getting the programs developed but have some ongoing issues to fine-tune. In previous chapters you have read about systemic processes, internal referral routing and processing, conversion rates, and so on. Within this chapter we will share a few examples from assessments and a few ideas on what to look for in studying the competition within the market.

COMPETITIVE ASSESSMENTS

This section could open with: "To mystery shop or not to shop, that is the question. Whether 'tis nobler to snoop or to suffer the slings and arrows of outrageous competition, to close perchance, to compete no more." While how you do it is your choice, it is absolutely imperative that you become intimately acquainted with your competition, so that you may see what the patient public sees. As referenced in Chapter 16 on assisted living, we have included a competitive assessment. This skilled and assisted living facility was aware that there were areas in which they possibly did not offer some services necessary to be competitive within the market; however, they also felt strongly that there were several areas that were strong points for them. We visited all of the competitors in the area and made suggestions on how the facility could position itself more strongly within the local market area.

COMPETITIVE ASSESSMENT—ASSISTED LIVING

Situation: The facility in a large metropolitan area has a well-established reputation for quality. The facility has been well positioned as a niche provider, with a private-pay clientele who, in the words of the executive director, "want the very best." Several providers have entered the market, and the executive director was interested in determining if the facility was positioned well compared with the other providers. The facility ownership was considering the need for some service enhancements and was interested in the public's perception of the facilities to choose from. We visited four competitors, and have included the tables on their services (pages 241-246).

Next we gave our brief assessment of the more important points of each facility.

Facility Impressions
Facility 3

Strengths:	Weaknesses:
Visually the nicest facility. Presents an initial view of costs, which may attract individuals to this facility over the client's facility.	Marketing director did not conduct effective tour; very condescending. No nursing care for residents with special needs. The

T A B L E 19-1

Facility Comparisons

	Issue/Area: First Impressions		
Facility 1	**Facility 2**	**Facility 3**	**Facility 4**
Setting—near shopping and thoroughfares, but set off the road	Concrete and commercial	On main thoroughfare, but set off the street; landscaped and quiet	Quiet, residential setting
Parking insufficient at healthcare entrance	Parking insufficient; "mystery shopper" was blocked in by another visitor	Plentiful parking	Biggest parking lot, with ample lighting
Smallest, most cluttered lobby; few chairs	The only facility not decorated in coral/rose shades; teal, blue, and beige	Hotel-like entrance; nine sets of business cards at front desk	Large and well lit, with small reception desk; furniture nice but not plush
Quickly greeted by well-informed receptionist	Quickly greeted by receptionist	Coffee service and newspapers in lobby	Receptionist an excellent marketer (is a resident)

Issue/Area: Miscellaneous

Facility 1	Facility 2	Facility 3	Facility 4
Recently purchased by Corporation Z; encouraged us to tour Facility No. 3 also	Have a lovely ice cream parlor with country store	Issues alert pendants to go around residents' necks	Entire continuum available
Have two two-bedroom suites, much larger than the regular sizes, with a shared living area	Spoke with six-year resident—very complimentary regarding staff; said food had improved and chef was now from hotel	Spoke with resident there since opening—very complimentary about food and staff	Building fifty-bed Alzheimer's unit
Thirty assisted-living suites	Nice courtyard	Lovely sunroom and courtyard	Only facility with two pull cords in bathrooms, one near toilet and one by shower
Does not allow coffeemakers but does allow microwave			
Cable TV	No cable TV	Cable TV	No cable TV

Issue/Area: Transportation

Facility 1	Facility 2	Facility 3	Facility 4
Provide transportation within a five-mile radius for doctor visits or shopping	Provide transportation within ten-mile radius for any hospital (except Hospital X) or place that one wants to shop	Provides transportation on predetermined routes only to nearby hospitals	Have van service daily to affiliated hospital and senior center
Residents must have someone accompany them as the service is "curb to curb" only	Will take and pick up resident anywhere in ten-mile radius on Tuesdays; resident must schedule ahead of time	Activities Department takes the van out on recreational outings	Provider service on Monday and Wednesday to Hospital Y
		Many residents keep their own cars	Regularly scheduled trips are for residents to go shopping, to the grocery, etc.

Issue/Area: Activities

Facility 1	Facility 2	Facility 3	Facility 4
Holds five to six activities per day during the week (among three floors)	Offers the most activities daily and a comparable schedule on weekends	No activities calendar available	Fewer activities than any other facility
Offers movie matinee on Sunday afternoons	Offers Saturday and Sunday drives		Promotes that activities are led mostly by residents

243

Issue/Area: Dining Areas

Facility 1	Facility 2	Facility 3	Facility 4
Dining room small; not as well-appointed as the surroundings	Large dining room, much like that in older, moderately priced hotel	Hotel-type dining room, hotel atmosphere	Elegant dining room
Table cloths, linen	Low, circular vinyl chairs	Choices in A.M. of Continental breakfast in one's room or hot breakfast in the dining room	Linen and china service
Crepe paper decorations	No tablecloths, no flowers	Lunch and dinner: two entrees with salad bar; other daily choices (sandwiches, salad plates)	Two entree choices at lunch and dinner
Two entree choices posted	Plastic placemats	Two seatings; elegant menu with two entrees displayed under glass; linen cloths, linen napkins, fresh flowers on tables	Menu is displayed daily and has very large type for residents
	Salad bar		

Issue/Area: Living areas, with fees

Facility 1	Facility 2	Facility 3	Facility 4
Monthly Rates:	Monthly rentals with add-on rates:	Four levels of care at add-on rates—see materials.	Efficiency A (456 sq. ft.) $1,940
Model A or B with 300 square feet is $2,350 per month	Efficiency (312 sq. ft.) $1,400	Space-only rates:	Efficiency B (540 sq. ft.) $2,080
Has two double suites available (two-bedroom with sandwich living space) for $2,500 per month	One bedroom (473 sq. ft.) $1,750	A Level 1 $1,990–$2,090 Level 2 $2,030–$2,130	One bedroom, one bath (624 sq. ft.) $2,630
Extras: Kitchenette with-two burner range, small refrigerator; private shower and bath	Best compact (hideaway) built in space for kitchenette with two-burner range and refrigerator; private baths and showers	B Level 1 $1,990–$2,090 Level 2 $2,150–$2,340	Two-burner range and small refrigerator, private bath and shower
		C Level 1 $2,050–$2,190 Level 2 $2,250–$2,390	
		D Level 1 $2,500–$2,600 Level 2 $2,700–$2,800	
		No range, although one may bring a small refrigerator to install in a built-in area; private bath and shower	

Issue/Area: Brochures and information packet

Facility 1	Facility 2	Facility 3	Facility 4
One 4-by-5-inch pocket folder; corporate piece with one page customized; business cards inserted	One 9-by-12-inch packet; teal and black on white inserts; business cards inserted	One 6-by-9-inch packet with full color and photos; corporate; customized, with local business cards and inserts	One 4-by-9-inch packet with full color photos and inserts
Inserts: selecting a healthcare center; name therapy; one customized sheet with photos, floor plans, etc.; services and amenities (rates); newsletter, activity calendar (includes name of the manager on duty for every weekend)	Inserts: menu; facility newsletter; monthly fee sheet; assisted-living services (rates); one 8-by-11 inch foldout; one general promo sheet	Inserts: services and amenities; floor plans; fee schedules; maps; corporate newsletter; little local focus	Inserts: activities calendar; rates; floor plans

Refer to list of services and amenities; many represent add-on fees.

client's facility can promote this care for people who may need extra assistance or who have a history of illness.

Facility 1

Strengths:
Purchased by another group; expect changes and improvements.

Weaknesses:
Not as elegant as expected or promoted.
While activity calendar appears to be full, it is for three floors.
Parking is insufficient at the healthcare center.
Poorest first impression of a lobby area.

Facility 2

Strengths:
Best activities calendar and transportation.
Affordable care with more assistance and services available.
Appears to be the best value.

Weaknesses:
Parking is horrendous.

Facility 4

Strengths:
The full continuum of care is offered on one campus.

Weaknesses:
No furniture is provided.
Residents must provide their own linens.
There is no crossover between dining for different levels of care as there is at the Client's facility.

We have included a few of the issues and areas of opportunity we identified for this facility based on the investigation conducted. It was our hope to share with them how the public could perceive their services in comparison with other providers and to offer considerations for improvements or enhancements.

Opportunities

Finding: Add-on charges initially represent some facilities' fees as lower than they are in reality. The Client's costs may appear even higher to casual or first-time inquiries, thus hindering further investigation.

Recommendation: Construct a sheet for admissions packet to emphasize the depth of services (i.e., value for monthly investment: furniture, linens, laundry, professional services, assistance, meals, etc.,) offered at the Client's facility, so that costs do not artificially appear higher in comparison to competitors.

Finding: Activities are a strong selling point for admissions within this service. However, several facilities appear to offer more activities than the client.

Recommendation: Consider creative ways to increase the number of activities by adding such features as more movies.

Finding: While no facility actually appears to have better food service than the client, others present it better by offering menus and visual presentations near the dining room. This is effective on tours. Facilities with lesser quality present better than the client. This may affect decisions.

Recommendation: Explore the possibility of better promotion, including inserting menus in admission/inquiry packets and offering one elegant display menu as others do.

Finding: Other facilities offer efficiency or one-bedroom apartments, in contrast to client's offerings of smaller areas (more like rooms than apartments).

Recommendation: Position client's rooms as "personal living areas" in the video and tours; revisit the appearance of "model rooms" within the facility to ensure that furniture is positioned for maximum open feeling. The large antiques are nice but tend to make areas appear smaller.

Finding: In reviewing inquiry data, effective tours appear to be the key to client admissions. When families tour they tend to admit. (Note that more than 96 percent of those touring admit.)

Recommendation: Encourage inquiries to tour, produce inquiry video, and conduct monthly tour in-service for managers as to depth of services, etc. Select a different manager every month to take the executive director on a tour and practice.

OUTPATIENT REHABILITATION POINTS OF INQUIRY

Many facilities are adding outpatient rehabilitation facilities to their continuums of care. The decision to focus on sports or industrial medicine or the geriatric population obviously depends upon the demographics of the area, the local industry, and the organization's patient population.

Whether the facility is established or still in the planning stages, it is important to know the competition. We include questions you may wish to incorporate into a check-off questionnaire for a more efficient visit and overview. You may also use this format to scrutinize your own facility and see how it measures up.

Outpatient Facility Profile

Accessibility:	Is the facility located on a main thoroughfare, a primary road or secondary road, or a one-way street?
Implications:	Is it difficult to get to? Will a prospective patient choose another provider instead, given these issues?
Signage:	Is there adequate signage? Would you have noticed it or passed it if you were visiting for the first time?
Implications:	Would you drive by it and choose another provider?

Surroundings:	Is the area commercial, a healthcare organization campus, freestanding, in a mall or an industrial park, or rural? Are there safety-perception issues?
Implications:	Will patients want to come here for treatment? Is it "safe" and convenient, or out of the way?
Exterior and Curb Appeal:	On driving up, what is the setting? Is it concrete, well manicured or in need of mowing, well landscaped or overgrown?
Implications:	What does it say about your facility and your care?
Parking:	What is the parking situation? Is there adequate parking? Is there a lot? Is there on-street parking? Is parking close to the door for those patients who may have mobility issues?
Implications:	Have we made it easy or difficult to be a patient here?
Lobby:	Is it inviting, or small and crowded? Is there an open window or a closed one? Is the receptionist readily available or hidden behind the frosted glass? Are there enough chairs, and how many are there? Does the lobby have welcoming accouterments (TV, soft music, magazines, etc.)?
Implications:	Do patients feel welcome? If they must wait are they occupied? If the receptionist is hidden, do patients feel ignored or like an intruder?
Decor:	Is it inviting and tasteful or does it appear to be leftovers from goodness knows where?
Implications:	Is it welcoming and comfortable or are the chairs instruments of torture? If it doesn't measure up to expectations, it reflects on the quality of care in the public's eyes.
Hours:	Hours are very important. Does the facility close during lunch? Does it have evening,

	early-morning, or weekend hours? Is it keeping away business or making it accessible? Can patients minimize time away from work or other responsibilities?
Services:	Industrial medicine, work conditioning, industrial preventative programs, drug testing, pain programs, physician services in occupational medicine, an internist, physiatrist, preemployment physicals. Comprehensive Outpatient Rehabilitation Programs (CORF). Therapy services (respiratory, physical therapy, occupational therapy, speech therapy, prosthetics, durable medical equipment. Other services (nursing, psychological, social services, medications, nutritional, and physician); pediatric services.
Implications:	Are services competitive in their depth or will patients be forced to leave to receive another component, thus encouraging them to leave the continuum and enter the competition's?
Staff:	How many and what type?
Implications:	Are there enough staff to take care of patients within every specialty, or will patients leave?
Payors:	Medicare, Medicaid, participation in managed care, insurances, workers' compensation.
Implications:	Will certain patients be better served elsewhere (not necessarily a negative)?
Rooms/ Services:	Are there exercise rooms, treatment rooms, offices, whirlpools, a large gym, swimming pool? What type of equipment is present?
Implications:	Again, depth of services and accommodations for a larger patient load or different types of patients.
Insurer and MD Communi- cations:	How often are reports sent to insurers, employers, and MDs? Are they verbal or written?

Implications: Is service provided to referral sources?
Lag Time   How quickly is the facility seeing
from Referral   patients who are referred? How long must
to Admissions: one wait?
Implications: This is related to staff and hours to some
                    extent. Are there enough staff to see
                    patients in a timely fashion or will they go
                    elsewhere to have their problems addressed
                    sooner. This is especially important to
                    employers and insurers.
Ownership: Who owns the venture?
Implications: Does there appear to be a built-in stream of
                    patients? If the facility is hospital based, will
                    it be taking your previous referral base?
Issues: Upcoming renovation, expansion of
                    services, new employees in specialties,
                    physician medical director, and so on.
Implications: New competitor information that one
                    needs to be aware of can be identified.

This is a start in determining what opportunities there are for your facility or what improvements can be made to be more successful in attracting patients.

FREESTANDING SKILLED FACILITY

As more and more hospitals expand their continuums of care, freestanding skilled facilities, acute rehabilitation centers, long-term care hospitals, and home health organizations are facing the challenges of diminishing referrals. An assessment was done for a freestanding skilled facility that had experienced a reduction in admissions to the Medicare unit when services had actually been expanded. The facility was located about one hour from a metropolitan area. The facility staff had been marketing. An inquiry, referral, and admissions assessment was performed, using the same type of approach as outlined in Chapter 11 on internal strategies to improve the continuum. We suspected that the facility's census problem was a combination of two situations: the small size of the local patient population pool and the marketing of the facility. It was our charge to determine specifically where opportunity lay to generate the desired level of census and to make recommendations on how to take advantage of that opportunity.

The facility had an assistant administrator who handled all admission functions and a Medicare nurse who coordinated care on the Medicare unit. We interviewed these individuals and the administrator to identify areas of opportunity. We also reviewed the inquiry and admission logbooks for the past two years to identify trends. Here we have included the interviews. As you read, relate this section to your previous readings regarding referral sources (immediate, intermediate, and long term) so that you may determine where the clients were in relation to where they needed to be. Make notes in the margins and compare your findings to ours.

Assistant Administrator Interview

Stated Job Responsibilities: She handles all outside marketing, events, MD offices, physician contacts, hospital social worker contacts, all paperwork of the "office manager."

Inquiry Process: She takes all inquiries.

Tours: She tries to conduct most of the tours.

Why do people choose your facility? "Because it is so clean. Everyone is nice and it makes a good first impression."

What marketing is involved in your role? Do you visit discharge planners and physicians? Hospital discharge planners—visits and takes something, such as notepads and brochures, muffins, fruit, cookies.

Physicians—This is harder to do. She does take something every now and then, but not very often. She gets to the offices about once per quarter. Plans to try more often. States that time is a problem.

What is the admission policy? The facility accepts patients seven days a week and twenty-four hours a day if the patients have their paperwork in order (state-mandated paperwork history and physical (H & P), lab, etc.).

Can you estimate the percentage of referrals coming from physicians, families, and discharge planning professionals?

Physicians	0%
Families	50%
Discharge planners	50%

Can you estimate the percentage of referrals from the nearby hospitals? Only a few patients, those with more intensive care needs, go into the metropolitan area for care. Local Hospital A accounts for virtually all of the referrals.

Do you have marketing meetings? Yes. They were held weekly. All department heads attend. They discuss issues, problems, and actual projects, which are completed on a twelve week marketing plan.

Tell me about some of the highlights of the marketing plan. Recently we purchased an outdoor sign, and we use it to publicize the resident and employee of the month, as well as to advertise events.

A representative goes to the local retirement center every Wednesday.

We send flower arrangements to the residents' churches and have gotten much positive press from the clergy for this, and we also have many new volunteers as a result."

(Note: The marketing plans for previous quarters were provided to us.)

Medicare Nurse Interview

Stated Job Responsibilities: Coordinates care for all of the Medicare Part A patients—admitting, audits, and monitoring patient progress. Obtains orders for Part B services and chairs team conference meetings once a week.

Why do people choose your facility? "During tours we stress how therapists are in the building with their own office and room. People also can see how many activities we have—it is very busy."

What hospitals refer to you the most? Local Hospital A, with a few from the metropolitan hospital 1.

What marketing is involved in your role? Do you visit discharge planners? Yes, once a week. She also goes to the retirement home once a week. She visits the hospital with teddy bears when a resident is admitted. When new patients are admitted, she goes to see some of the physicians to give them the facility's goals and to explain skilled and rehab units.

What skilled services do you offer? IV antibiotics, therapy, Ventilator care (only ones in area to do so), Rehab and respiratory, and New G tubes. (Patients are transferred out for transfusions)

Administrator Interview

What are some of the census issues you face? The social workers share patients among all of the local Medicare units. This dilutes our census. The census is ninety to ninety-five. Medicare patients have declined from eighteen to ten. Remodeling is in progress, which affects census.

What about the facility's reputation? "The facility has a reputation for good patient care. Two social workers just came in and said that we give the 'best care,' and soon we will have a beautiful building."

What can you tell me about the staff? The director of nursing (DON) has been here for three years, and is to move to be the care plan/MDS nurse. The new DON (also a native of the area) will start soon. The Medicare nurse works well with physicians after working ten to twelve years at the local hospital.

How do you sell the services—what are the strong points? On longevity of the staff and low turnover.

How effective are tours? "We usually admit prospective patients if they or their family members tour. We stress central heat and air in each room and the new call-light system. We introduce them to members of the marketing team (department heads), who have all been here at least five years. We have conducted certified tour guide training for nurse's aides and in-serviced them on telephone usage."

Tell me about your marketing efforts. We participate in all community events, from the chili cook-off to the college events (take an ad in the paper supporting). We have candy jars all over town in businesses, pharmacies, lumberyards, MD offices, etc. At Christmas we deliver calendars. We have an ongoing twelve-week marketing plan. Food services goes to the nutrition center with homemade items and brochures. We take blood pressures once a week at the retirement home. Every Fourth of July we hold a cookout and prepare about 400 hot dogs and 300 hamburgers, we invite each doctor's office and people from the hospitals, as well as the ambulance workers, police officers, and firefighters. We box up lunches for the units at the hospitals and send them over with a watermelon. The administrator, Medicare nurse, and assistant administrator go to hospitals at least once a week, sometimes two times, just to drop in. We have a bold listing, but no yellow pages ad. We recognize a "doctor of the quarter." We do not generally take out ads in the newspaper, but will send in a story about once a week on the resident and employee of the month and publicize special events (such as Nursing Home Week). If the high school or college does a promo item, will take ads.

FACILITY IMPRESSIONS

STRENGTHS

The facility is clean and nice; it makes a good first impression.

Discharge planners at the local hospital are visited about once a week, sometimes twice (note the hospital does not have a skilled unit).
It does conduct regular marketing meetings.

The facility has a twelve-week marketing plan.
The facility has established reputation for good care and has staff-community ties.
Therapy is a selling point during tours. Emphasizes the onsite team, therapy space, and office area.
When new patients are admitted, staff visits some physicians to educate them on skilled and rehab units and to give them patients' goals.

WEAKNESSES

Once-a-quarter contact with physicians is insufficient to change the current physician referral pattern—approximately 0 percent.
Local hospital comprises 99 percent of all of the facility referrals. The significance of this is that census in the facility must follow that of the local hospital.
The marketing plan appears to be events centered instead of one-on-one-contact centered with events supporting (although we do understand the importance of events in smaller towns).
The metropolitan market with a number of hospitals appears to be virtually untapped; it has potential for the more complex patients that the facility desires.

Longevity of staff.

Tours are very effective. Tour
training was conducted for
staff at all levels.

The competition reportedly
conducts little marketing
compared with the client
facility.

There is a good twenty-four
hours-a-day-seven-day-a-
week admission policy.

The administrator is astute
about marketing.

The facility uses newspapers
well.

The facility has established a
good community profile
through good patient care
and effective public relations.

There appears to be a team
effort in the marketing approach.

FACILITY OBSERVATIONS

Finding: There is opportunity for increased focus on one-to-one
contact with physicians. Fifty percent of referrals are driven
by social workers, with fifty percent driven by families. The fam-
ily-driven referrals have a very high conversion rate, reflecting the
efficiency of the process. Unfortunately, the social work referrals
are often to multiple providers. The conversion rate decreases, as
does the efficiency of the process. Increasing the physician-driven
referrals would most likely increase Medicare census and the conversion rate, because physician directed referrals generally have a
higher conversion rate. This is particularly true in smaller towns.

Recommendation: Consider developing a plan to regularly (once
a month) call on physician offices in the area (with different

tools to be developed—case studies, admission/discharge notification, etc.). Consider doctor's office staff events.

Finding: The local hospital refers 99 percent of all patients referred. The census in the facility depends solely upon this hospital creating a situation where census trends will follow those at the hospital. Consistent marketing appears to be conducted at the local hospital, but none is conducted at the nearby metropolitan hospitals.

Recommendation: Consider marketing to the nearby metropolitan hospitals once a month so that outmigration of the most-ill patients (complex patients) will be recaptured and returned to your facility. In this way the census will be more than what is garnered from the local facility and not wholly dependent on census trends from the local hospital.

Finding: The marketing plan appears to be events centered (there is only one physician/social worker reference). More emphasis on referral sources needs to be in place to drive referrals from areas other than the public (long-term census builders).

Recommendation: Consider developing an ongoing focus on social workers, nurses on hospital units, therapists in the acute care hospital, and physicians and physician's office staffs to shift major emphasis to actual referral sources. Use events and community activities to finalize the choice; you will already have strong recognition and an established reputation. Community involvement is important, especially in smaller areas, but the facility is very likely to be able to shift some resources and efforts to referral sources without adverse affect. If any public relations, survey, or quality issues arise, the public effort should shift and increase for situational needs.

Finding: The facility has built goodwill and an awareness within the community. This is an excellent basis on which to now move further to broaden the awareness of the complexity of patients accepted, the transitional nature to home, and the facility as more than a nursing home. If social workers are dividing up referrals "fairly" within the area, this should help drive preferences through awareness that this facility is capable of more complex care.

Recommendation: Consider shifting some resources for community public relations to developing community education programs to focus the area on the complexity of care; "How to Choose a Nursing Facility," for example.

DISCUSSION OF THE ANALYSIS

As you can see, our focus is to increase direct, one-to-one educational contacts with primary and secondary referral sources. With weekly and monthly call-rotation schedules, the staff can see what they need to accomplish and become more focused on generating referrals and converting them to census.

The focus here is 90 percent sales, augmented by 10 percent public relations (events, case studies, patient stories, etc.). The public relations is necessary because of public attitudes toward "nursing homes." Our impetus is to shift the paradigm to "nursing and rehabilitation centers" and to educate the community on the expertise of this client facility. The work with hospital-based referral sources necessitates conducting one-to-one contacts and must replace a "goody giving" mentality for both cost-effectiveness and message marketing.

It appears to us that the administration of the facility is to be commended for optimizing internal staff resources for the marketing effort. We especially admired the investment in training all staff to perform tours. Remember, the facility presented well, and many individuals were likely to tour at off-hours. Therefore, the ability for any employee to conduct a quality tour was imperative.

Clearly, the challenge is to take the effort to the next level by increasing *continuous* contact with physicians and their office staffs and educating the referral sources and the public regarding the level of services provided, as well as the transition of short-stay patients from the hospital to home. Another challenge is to capture patients who outmigrate for care to the nearby metropolitan area. We provided specific and detailed ideas on how to begin to work toward these goals in a marketing plan for the client. Many of the projects suggested were included in several different sections of this book and creatively modified to meet the clients' needs.

IDENTIFYING AREAS OF CONCERN AND POTENTIAL STRATEGIES

Often clients bring issues to us and ask for recommendations on strategies to address the problems. What follows are a few ideas on some of the most often-asked questions.

ISSUES	SIGNIFICANCE	APPROACHES
History of incidents, or survey difficulties.	Elephants never forget. There will always be those who will choose not to refer and those who will be long-term targets for changing their referral patterns.	Public Relations: Showcase the facility, especially if it is aesthetically pleasant, with public seminars and events; residents and families should participate. Call on referral sources to honestly address past problems and current facility improvement or those in progress. Begin a family reference network (Refer to Chapter 20). Submit human interest success stories in the newspaper. Prepare staff bio sheets (Refer to Chapter 20). If possible, announce every new employee in the newspaper. If the facility has a deficiency-free evaluation or is accredited or commended, put it in the paper and display an announcement or banner.

ISSUES	SIGNIFICANCE	APPROACHES
Facility does not "show" well.	Competition may present better. Many families cannot judge medical capabilities. The entire focus is developing a facility that people will select for *their* *care*, not on its looks. You must position the facility as being superior to others in town on the basis of service delivery.	Conduct a competitive analysis to share the competitive issues objectively. Determine if subtle changes can be economically made. Focus the facility on cleanliness. Focus the staff on a service mentality. Conduct extensive tour training for the facility admissions coordinator and the entire management staff to emphasize a sales mentality and skills, not frills, during tours. Get employees involved on tours. Offer clinical information on tours and in packets. Print supplemental materials to focus on services offered and experience/expertise of those on staff. Erect a success board display in the front lobby *(consents must be on file)*. Include success stories, notes, and photos.

ISSUES	SIGNIFICANCE	APPROACHES
The provider has census, (patient load), but patients are not the optimal population desired.	Therapists and nurses desire the challenge of these types of patients. Facility-plan projections are not being met. Note—building confidence in the staff, as well as service development and promotion to the public, may be a large portion of this effort. If this is the case, refer to techniques listed in the first section of this chart, "History of incidents."	Perform a DRG study to identify the exact types of patients within the population pool. Actively market for these patients. Conduct an internal analysis and logbook review to determine if the problem is referrals or conversion of referrals to admissions. Address specifically. Develop case studies and brochures on services delivery. Conduct in-service education for physicians' staffs and hospital-based referral sources. Have therapists and nurses visit their acute care peers. Educate admissions coordinator, marketing intake coordinator, or receptionist to conduct focused tours and handle inquiries more effectively. Procure free brochures from organizations on these diagnoses to include in packets and develop diagnoses sheets in patient packets.

ISSUES	SIGNIFICANCE	APPROACHES
		Conduct one-to-one referral development with appropriate tools.
		Consider community education to focus on complex services offered.
The admissions or marketing coordinator, receptionist, or intake coordinator is new or not functioning at an optimal level.	Is unable or unwilling to sell appropriate services or target the right type of patients.	Become his or her "best" friend within the facility.
		Teach about the services offered and provide a cheat sheet book to use on the phone.
		Offer to participate or take over a tour when the employee gets to the clinical areas.
		Provide sales and tour training, with opportunities to practice the skills.
		Provide information about diagnoses and therapy/clinical interventions.
		Offer to go on calls or tag along to meet acute care hospital referral sources.
		Offer to go out on assessments with the employee to screen patients.

CONCLUSION

We hope that this chapter has provided insight into appraising one's facility and processes, as well as the importance of being familiar with the promotional aspects and features of the competition. Internal assessment is the first step in identifying opportunities for improvement. Oftentimes it is internal systems that interfere with an organization's success, not the external factors. Through internal assessment we can objectively determine process issues that we can address to improve effectiveness in all areas, not just marketing. Many times our work begins with marketing issues but leads us to the operations arena because the two are inextricably intertwined. External factors are ever-present. Yet somehow, we can be blissfully ignorant of them and their effect on our daily success. As we have stated, marketing management must go beyond some of our traditional boundaries and delve into other areas to see the organization as a whole, identify issues, and let opportunity meet preparedness.

20 CHAPTER

The Marketer's Toolbox

Builders often say, "You can build anything with the right tools." We in marketing have supplied our hospitals with tools for years. Whether the need was a brochure or advertisement, marketing was called. The sales force and internal staff also need tools—in this case, props for presentations. We will include many such tools within this chapter.

If you have been in healthcare for any length of time or have recently visited your physician, you have seen pharmaceutical reps with their detail bags. These people are easy to spot. They are usually the best-dressed people in the office, with the biggest bags and a never-ending stream of giveaways. In healthcare, this is the one approach that we prefer not to take.

We recommend that your field marketers dress conservatively and deliver clinically oriented items that distinguish them from detail people. This recommendation stems from the classic sales-training directive to "never outdress your customer." In the past, one was more likely to see office staff in uniforms. With the advent of a more casual lifestyle at home and work, we are seeing more and more staff members moving to street clothes, sometimes covered with a lab coat. If the field rep is a clinician, we recommend wearing a lab coat with a name tag or monogram to include the clinical title. This way the field rep is positioned as a clinical problem solver, not a salesperson. Nothing is more degrading to a rep than to be told, "I'm sorry he doesn't see vendors" or "He only sees vendors on certain days." I've been there and, believe me, it is about as appealing to a clinician as being likened to a snake-oil salesman.

There are a number of excellent sales training books on the market to be required reading for your reps. A few tricks of the trade follow.

GETTING AN APPOINTMENT

Don't bother to phone. Think of those solicitation calls at your home, when you are busy or in the middle of dinner. You've probably perfected the ten-second hang-up, as most people have. We suggest using cold calls to set up appointments. It is a lot harder to say no to a smiling face at the window with an appointment book than to a voice over the phone. Ask what day of the week or what certain time would be best and go from there.

The best reason to go in person is that it is one more contact in your mission to schedule referral relationships. Conversely, there are reps who never cold-call, even for appointments. See what works best in your area and go with it.

Don't Overlook the Importance of the Office Staff

When I've opened new territories, I have focused first on the office staff, not the physician. They can invariably tell you details about the practice, what types of patients they see, where the physician practices, where he or she refers, the payor mix, and so on. In sales lingo they are called "gatekeepers" or "influencers." Who speaks informally with families about different healthcare providers? The physician office staffs do, and they are a tremendous referral source. They are a fountain of knowledge about the practice and can provide an entry to the physician's inner sanctum. Conversely, they can provide information that indicates that this physician doesn't belong on the contact rotation list. In working with these staffers, the Golden Rule applies. Treat these people as you'd like to be treated. Don't send a thank-you note only to the physician; also thank the person who got you in the door. How often do we get thanked for little things in life? Ask yourself. Some of my best friendships have stemmed from referral relationships.

The highest courtesy to an office staff is to be able to leave graciously if the office is busy, then plan to return another day. Please note that we do not advocate just saying, "I'll come back another day." Close the call by saying (with your appointment book open at the window), "I can see that things are really busy here today. Could we schedule another day for me to return? Your patients are more important and it looks like everyone could be late going home as it is." Nine times out of ten the office staffer will appreciate your understanding and schedule another day. When you return on that day, refer to the particulars of the previous visit and you'll likely be seen in a timely fashion.

CASE STUDY

I was conducting sales training for a corporation and was familiar with all of the reps. One in particular did not seem to be very successful, judging by reports about his success. I was looking forward to the role-play section of the training, where the rep was to call on the office staff to determine the quality of his calls. It became very clear to me where the issue most likely lurked when, after just a few seconds of pleasantries, he stated that he only wanted to talk to the doctor. The effect would have been equivalent to saying, "I don't want to talk to you since you're not important. I want to see the doctor, who is important." That will no doubt cost relationships and referrals.

TOOLS

Once in the door, conduct the call and be certain to introduce your tools last. If you give them to the target early or during the call, it's only human nature that your contact will focus on reading and not on what you are saying. The whole focus of the call—to ask questions and to learn and share information—is hindered if the target is reading rather than speaking with you. Hold your tools until the conclusion of the conversation. Leave them with the office staff, or use them as a reason to return, so the individual can focus on the conversation and not on reading your brochure.

Tools are the props for our marketing calls. They are our reason for speaking with someone, and they speak for us when we are not there. Therefore, it is important that they have the ability to speak well for us and convey the desired message in a concise fashion. The look as well as the message is important. The following are a few examples of tools.

Program Communications—"Fax Commercials"

We include (on pages 269–272) a few sample sheets of what we call "fax commercials." These are 8½-by-11-inch sheets, usually on program letterhead. The top half of the sheet notifies the physician's office of the admission or discharge status of a patient. This is to improve communication and also to make the physician aware of such issues as room changes. I saw a hospital-based specialty unit use this tool very well after a key physician became angry when he came onto the unit and couldn't find his patient who had been transferred!

The bottom half of the admission sheet details the types of patients who are appropriate for the program. This should be able to be quickly scanned. Remember, we only have a few seconds to get the message across. The bottom half of the discharge sheet is about how to make a referral. It is more likely that you will generate another referral on the heels of a successful discharge. These messages can be done tastefully and ideally should be changed every few months so they will be read. This is also a perfect place to introduce new program staff and to make other announcements. Be creative with the message.

TEAM CONFERENCE NOTES OR PATIENT STATUS LETTERS

The format for team conference notes is usually one 8½-by-11-inch page, single sided, with the same typeface as the facility logo, and often on program or facility stationery.

The goal is to create a communication tool directed at physicians to promote the program while simultaneously conveying the progress of the patient. In many areas, specialty programs can be perceived as competing with physician practices instead of augmenting them. This communication tool is effective in subtly reinforcing the role of the patient's physician in any specialty program.

The notes usually take the form of an outline to be filled in by hand (or typed) and delivered either in person or by fax to the physician. The report briefly identifies areas of progress and also identifies those areas remaining to be addressed during the next phase of treatment. It educates the physician regarding the patient's plan of care and

(Program Letterhead)

Notification of Patient Beginning Outpatient Cardiac Rehab

Dr. _____ ,
Thank you for referring your patient, _____ , to the outpatient cardiac rehab program. The patient was seen for an initial visit on *(date)*. As the patient progresses through treatment, we will be providing brief updates to your office for the patient's file.

_____ , Program Director

Program Structure
- Patients must be clinically stable
- A twelve-week, thirty-six-session program, with three one-hour sessions per week
- Monitored exercise
- Supplemental education on the cardiac condition provided by nurse educator
- Specially trained professional staff including nurses, dietitians, and exercise physiologists

Eligibility
- Medicare patients must meet stated requirements: MI within twelve months, CABG or angina. Thirty-six sessions are allowed in the patient's lifetime.
- Only a subsequent MI or CABG will renew eligibility.
- Many insurance plans provide coverage. We will work with patients to verify coverage.

(Program Letterhead)

Notification of Patient Discharge from Cardiac Rehab

Dr. _____ ,

Your patient, _____ , has been discharged from the program. The patient did complete/did not complete the program. The summary of the patient's progress will be forwarded to you for your files.

Please note: If the patient did not complete the program and would like to resume the program in the future, we will work with you to attempt to facilitate this.

_____ , Program Director

Referral Process

Cardiac rehab is a physician-referred service provided by (name of hospital) as part of the continuum of care within the community. Our goal is to provide a service to help the individual return to a level of more independent functioning, and prevent recidivism.

Simply write a prescription for cardiac rehab or have a member of your staff phone (phone number).

We accept Medicare, insurance, and managed care patients.

Notification of Patient Beginning Physical Therapy Program

Dr. _____,

Thank you for referring your patient, _____, for physical therapy at *(name of hospital)*. This patient was seen for the initial visit on *(date)*. As the patient progresses through treatment, we will provide brief updates to your office for your files. We will phone your office to schedule your patient's follow-up visit upon completion of the therapy.

Signed, *(department representative, title)*

Therapy Services Provided by *(name of hospital)*

Physical therapy is a physician-referred service, concerned with the restoration of function and reduction of disability following an acute episode of illness, exacerbation of a more chronic disease process, an injury, or the loss of a body part. The goal is to help the individual return to an optimal level of functioning to allow greater independence or to reduce the burden on caregivers.

Program Features

Evaluation	Balance and coordination
Transfer training	Mobility (walking, stair climbing)
Gait training	Range of motion
Modalities (hot and cold)	Wheelchair mobility management
Wound care	Equipment assessment

Muscle strength and general conditioning
Training patients in the use of orthotics and prosthetics
Mobility with assistive devices (cane, quad cane, crutches, walker)

Types of patients often referred for physical therapy may include: Orthopedic conditions (postsurgical, arthritis, and amputee), neurological (Parkinson's, CVA, etc.), diabetes, postsurgical or complicated recovery patients, and diabetic/wound care.

Notification of Patient Discharge
From Physical Therapy Program

Dr. _____ ,
Your patient, _____ , was discharged from the physical therapy program at *(name of hospital)* on *(date)*. The summary of the patient's progress will be forwarded to your office for your files. The patient's follow-up appointment with you has been scheduled through *(first name)* of your office staff for *(day, date, time)*. Thank you for referring this patient and allowing us to augment your continuum of care.

Signed, *(therapy representative, title)*

Referral Process:

Physical therapy is a physician-referred service provided by *(name of hospital)* as part of the continuum of care within the local community. Our goal is to provide quality services to help the individual attempt to return to a higher level of functioning.

Simply write a prescription for physical therapy or have a member of your staff phone *(phone number)*.

We accept Medicare, insurance, and many managed care patients.

also specific treatment modalities. It can be completed by a single member of the treatment team either at a client's regularly scheduled session, team conferences, or upon discharge. Two sample formats from an inpatient geropsych unit appear on pages 274 and 275.

You may consider designing and purchasing a rubber stamp that will say "Physician Office Chart Copy." We encourage field reps to deliver these in person, stamped with the big red letters in the right upper corner. Many times when you bring these reports into the office and request a moment to discuss it with the physician, you find your-self escorted into the physician's office. If it is important to you it soon becomes important to other people.

THE PATIENT/RESIDENT SATISFACTION SURVEY

There is perhaps no more powerful marketing tool than the patient satisfaction survey. Yet of all of the tools at a facility's disposal, it is the least used. Consider that many providers, from surgicenters and physicians' offices to hospitals (and the individual programs within), distribute surveys. Generally they may be summarized, with a brief memo from a marketing director, and copied to multiple executives within the system to simultaneously point fingers or congratulate. Afterward they all too often seem to be relegated to some dusty binder or file for an accrediting body to review. This is not the way to maximize scarce marketing resources. Ideally, you should follow up on these surveys (whether favorable or unfavorable) with a phone call and a short note. This is the opportunity to convey and explain points to the consumer. While these conversations must be managed, they represent an untapped opportunity.

Favorable responses are the best advertisements, more effective than any one ad can develop. We encourage programs to deliver these marketing tools to physicians' offices monthly to demonstrate positive responses from patients. Positive responses allow referral-source reinforcement and support for the referral decision, and encourage a comfort level for future referrals. Some readers may cringe at the thought of delivering the unfavorable report card. In classic sales methods we identify the delivery and ensuing discussion of the unfavorable response as a perfect sales opportunity. That is, delivering the bad news with the same reliability as the good news positions the provider as the individual or facility with the integrity to discuss and rectify their own

(Hospital or Program Letterhead)

January 3, 199X

William Gooddoctor
1234 S. Penn #101
Your City, USA 11111

Dear Dr. Gooddoctor:

This letter is to inform you of Annie Beensick's discharge from Renaissance, the Geriatric Mental Health Unit at Name of Health Center on December 27, 199X.

As you know, Annie Beensick was admitted to the geropsych unit on November 9, 199X. She was experiencing visual and auditory persecutory hallucinations and delusions. Her final diagnosis was degenerative dementia of the Alzheimer's type.

Social Services reported that Ms. Beensick made significant progress in her physical and emotional functioning during her stay. Ms. Beensick's hallucinations did not follow her to the hospital and she was able to refocus so that she functioned exceedingly well within the therapeutic milieu on the unit.

Occupational Therapy reported that upon discharge, Ms. Beensick was able to make positive self statements and to view herself as being more capable to deal with her individual needs. Ms. Beensick was also able to appropriately interact with peers and staff members in a caring manner and she developed a more positive attitude about coping with her life changes and adapting to new situations.

At discharge, Ms. Beensick was on the following medications:

Humulin N 65 units every AM, 30 units every PM
Cardizem CD 180 mg   Lanoxin 0.25 mg
Relefen 500 mg   Haldol 2 mg
Cogentin 1 mg   Fibercon

I hope this synopsis of care has informed you of pertinent information concerning Ms. Beensick. We appreciate the opportunity to work with you and your patient population. If we may be of further assistance to you, please do not hesitate to call us at XXX-XXXX.

Sincerely,

(Name)
(Title)
Geriatric Mental Health Unit

(Hospital or Program Letterhead)

April 12, 199X

Dr. Glenn Wellness
1234 S.W. 59th St. #104
Your City, USA 11112

Dear Dr. Wellness:

This is to inform you that Paul Wassick has been discharged from the Geriatric Mental Health Unit at Name of Health Center. He was admitted on March 16, 199X and discharged April 5, 199X. Paul was admitted depressed, experiencing paranoia and "seeing things in his food." He was admitted from the skilled nursing unit (SNU) where he was recovering from a wound dehiscence.

During neuropsych testing Paul revealed that he had fears related to hallucinations. Paul reported that his fears and issues of passivity were related to his marital situation. He attended, participated, and verbalized positive changes in perception and coping skills during his group therapies. He was able to acknowledge changes needed in his relationship with his spouse and need for caring for himself. Paul has been able to return to his volunteer work here at the hospital since his discharge.

Discharge recommendations were for Mr. Wassick to follow up with Dr. Van Good at 9:00 a.m. on April 6.

We appreciate the opportunity to work with you and your patient population. If we may be of further assistance to you, please do not hesitate to call us at XXX-XXXX.

Sincerely,

(Name)
(Title)
Geriatric Mental Health Unit

dirty-laundry issues. Isn't it preferable to apprise a physician of a patient's issues before his or her four- to six-week follow-up appointment? This gives the physician a "heads up" regarding the stay and the opportunity to clarify issues. This is also the opportunity to give a note to the physician regarding follow-up that has occurred with the individual by phone or letter. A sample format provided by a skilled and assisted-living facility is shown in Figure 20–1. Remember as you develop the survey tool that it should be easy to respond to and have sufficient areas for open comments.

DIAGNOSIS AND DISCIPLINE SHEETS

In addition to free brochures available through groups such as the Arthritis Foundation and many others, diagnosis and discipline sheets can be an effective way to promote continuum services and educate the public and referral sources at the same time (see pages 278–279). These are simple 8½-by-11-inch sheets that include:

- Basic information about the disease or condition
- A description of the approach to care, that is, the programmatic features (not just a service listing but more a description of what and why)
- Program results—why should the individual consider this care and how it should benefit them.
- Alternately, you can use discipline specific treatment sheets, such as our sample sheets, on pages 280 and 281, regarding occupational therapy for the psychogeriatric patient.

CASE STUDY

The most effective tour I have ever taken at a skilled facility included diagnosis sheets effectively used to sell me on the facility's capabilities. I toured a skilled facility in Tennessee that was built and promoted as a rehabilitation center and never promoted as a skilled facility. Even though there were other skilled facilities in the area, they were considered to be nursing homes, not rehabilitation centers. As I toured with the marketing director, we stopped in the therapy area. An occupational therapist asked a few questions regarding my (fictitious) patient. As we discussed the stroke patient in question, she went to the file and gave me a number of sheets regarding stroke and stroke

---

HOW ARE WE DOING?

Please rate the following:

1	2	3	4	5
bad	poor	average	good	superb

					UPON ADMISSION/Leasing
☐	☐	☐	☐	☐	Paperwork explained and questions answered
☐	☐	☐	☐	☐	Condition of living space (walls, paint, doors, etc.)
☐	☐	☐	☐	☐	Cleanliness
☐	☐	☐	☐	☐	Cleanliness of facility
☐	☐	☐	☐	☐	FRIENDLINESS/HELPFULNESS OF STAFF:
☐	☐	☐	☐	☐	Nursing assistant/Orderly/Attendant,
☐	☐	☐	☐	☐	Nurse,
☐	☐	☐	☐	☐	Housekeeper,
					SINCE ADMISSION/Leasing
☐	☐	☐	☐	☐	Quality of care
☐	☐	☐	☐	☐	Friendliness of staff
☐	☐	☐	☐	☐	Cleanliness of living space
☐	☐	☐	☐	☐	Cleanliness of facility
☐	☐	☐	☐	☐	Quality/taste of meals
☐	☐	☐	☐	☐	Appearance/presentation of meals
☐	☐	☐	☐	☐	Personal laundry services
☐	☐	☐	☐	☐	Proper and homelike environment
☐	☐	☐	☐	☐	Services rendered as explained

Would you recommend this facility to others?   Yes ☐   No ☐

How could we make a resident's stay better? _____

_____

_____

Comments: _____

_____

Thank you for your time.   Signature Optional

Figure 20–1. Sample survey

care. As I later reviewed the sheets in detail, I could see that the materials had been developed and provided through the American Occupational Therapy Association. I remembered how difficult it was when my father had his stroke. At the time, with ten years of healthcare experience to my credit, I had no knowledge about strokes. I knew without a doubt that if I had been looking

Diagnosis Sheet Sample
Services for Persons With Arthritis

The Condition: Arthritis is a disease that affects the joints. It causes pain and decreased mobility, and it may affect other parts of the body. There is no cure for arthritis, which means it is very important for persons with arthritis to receive proper treatment and learn techniques that will enable them to best manage their condition.

Our Approach to Care: Because symptoms and difficulties can vary from individual to individual, we tailor specific care plans to the needs of patients. An evaluation is begun upon admission and the entire team (physician, nurses, physical and occupational therapists, social workers, psychologists, and therapeutic recreation/activity specialists) work with the patient to move toward goals that have been mutually set.

Goals for Your Program May Include:

- Joint-protection techniques: By mastering joint-protection techniques, individuals can learn how to use their joints more safely and perhaps alleviate further stress to the joints.

- Energy conservation techniques: By becoming adept at energy conservation techniques the individual may increase his or her endurance and maintain the balance of activity and rest.

- Increased independence with the activities of daily living: By working with occupational therapists, you will learn to use assistive devices in bathing, dressing, and grooming. For many, use of these handy tools can diminish reliance on others for some daily tasks.

- Increased mobility: Our physical therapists will work with you to maximize your mobility.
- Home evaluation: Our therapists will visit your home to identify areas of concern or necessary modifications. Your therapy will be tailored to the challenges that you face in your own environment and the goals for your return to more independent daily living.
- Arthritis education: Our nurses are available to assist you in learning more about the disease process so that you can be empowered by information and develop methods of living more successfully within the limits of the arthritis condition.
- Role of the patients and their support team: Patients become active participants in the rehabilitative process, supported by friends and family who may be involved in treatment and education.

How to Make a Referral: While anyone may initiate a referral, admission is by physician order only. If you believe that you or someone you know could benefit from rehabilitative services please phone our program director, *(name)*, at *(phone number)*. A screening assessment will be conducted free of charge. Rehabilitation services are covered by Medicare and many managed care plans if patients meet established criteria.

Occupational Therapy for the Psychogeriatric Patient

Occupational Therapists provide mental health services to geriatric patients with a variety of diagnoses which include:

Major Depression	Chronic psychiatric disease
Delirium	Substance abuse
Organic Mental Syndromes	Primary degenerative dementia of the Alzheimer's type and other dementias

Occupational Therapists assess the individual's functional capacities, plan appropriate treatment and make recommendations to other services taking into consideration age-related changes in physical functioning and cognition. Areas frequently assessed include:

Cognition	Need for Day Treatment
Self Care	Home Management
Task Performance	Community Living Skills
Time Management/Leisure	Independent Living Skills
Interpersonal Skills	Physical Functioning
Safety Awareness	Social Skills
Behaviors reflecting social norms, values, and customs	Life Satisfaction

Occupational Therapy for the psychogeriatric patient may include group or individual sessions on topics such as:

Reality Orientation	Self Care
Sensorimotor Integration	Community Living Skills
Retirement Planning	Social Skills
Home Management Skills	

Occupational Therapy techniques may include use of sensory activities, memorabilia, physical activity, adaptive equipment, educational resources and simulated or real life tasks that are purposeful and help the patient achieve the highest possible level of functioning. Specific goals, always developed in collaboration with the client may include:

- improving independence in activities of daily living
- improving safety awareness
- increasing leisure skills and purposeful use of time
- increasing or maintaining physical functioning
- increasing use of adaptive or compensatory techniques for declines in physical and cognitive skills
- successfully integrating life experiences

Goals for Occupational Therapy provided to the patient in the inpatient unit might include:

- assisting in stabilizing behaviors during an acute episode
- providing patient performance data to the treatment team
- observing and reporting on the patient's performance in response to medication
- improving patient performance in areas where deficits interfere with return to the least restrictive environment
- assisting in discharge planning
- evaluating for reentry and other community programs

Occupational therapy is dedicated to helping individuals gain the highest possible degree of functional independence in the tasks of daily life.

Occupational therapists hold bachelors or masters degrees and occupational therapy assistants are trained at the associated degree level. Occupational therapy education includes a broad range of course work that emphasizes the social, emotional, and psychological implications of illness and injury. Occupational therapy practitioners must complete supervised clinical internships in a variety of health care settings and are required to pass a national certification examination.

for a rehabilitation provider, I would have chosen this one. I have taken literally hundreds of tours and this is the only facility that has offered me diagnostic information. I believe that families touring appreciate this information. It can make the difference in their selection of a provider, as well as providing an invaluable service.

INDIVIDUAL PATIENT CASE STUDIES

To build your own case study, follow the templates (see pages 284–285) and these guidelines to produce a double sided 3 panel brochure.

1. Select the best patient for illustration purposes:
   - The best outcome: (return to home, greater independence within an alternative setting, better able to manage chronic condition, etc.)
   - What level of complexity you want to show (depth of services, etc.)
   - Specific diagnoses and complications
   - Which physician(s) you want to market to
   - What insurer you are trying to appeal to

2. The Look: Of course, your case study should resemble your system's current printed materials. However, there are many options for producing a cost-effective tool. There are companies that produce blank paper ("shells") in different colors, formats, and styles. These inexpensive "shells" conveniently go through printers so that you can produce tools quickly and cost effectively. You can have bells and whistles on a budget.

3. Style
   - Avoid abbreviations
   - Be concise—your case study has a better chance of being read
   - Use lay language, not medicalspeak, if for other audiences than physicians
   - Take nothing for granted: There are individuals who have no concept of what some interventions are all about—for example, occupational therapy and physiatry. Occupational therapy has to do with whatever one does that occupies their time. Physiatrists specialize in physical medicine and rehabilitation, but some individuals have mistaken the specialty for other areas of medicine.

CASE STUDY

I was with a representative of an acute rehab hospital years ago in a rural area of the South. The rep, a registered nurse, was calling on an older primary-care physician. She was focusing on augmenting care of patients, not losing them to another physician, and was very clear to mention several times that the hospital had a physiatrist as a medical director. She was very proud that the facility had secured the services of a physiatrist for their more rural area and promoted it quite heavily. The physician became noticeably and progressively more agitated as the call progressed, finally pushing his chair back from the desk and throwing his hands up into the air, saying, "Lady, I don't know why I should refer patients to you and I don't know why you have a foot doctor as your medical director." The moral of the story: never take for granted the knowledge level of the target.

CONTINUUM OF CARE CASE STUDY PRESENTATIONS

While the lunchtime educational series for physicians may have been in hospitals' repertoires for many years, the continuum case study takes the concept a step further. Many tumor conferences included the oncologist or surgeon discussing the patient, the radiologist sharing diagnostics, the pathologist reporting findings, and the oncologist or radiation oncologist discussing treatment and current status. These conferences generally presented a fine picture of the patient through the first steps of the continuum but did not show the entire continuum of services provided to the patient. A full-continuum case study can be a very successful mechanism.

It works best when the presenters are all physicians. Depending upon the hospital's space and climate, the case study may be presented only to physicians or to all interested employees. The continuum of care case study can work for all components of the continuum of care. Following are some critical points:

1. *Select the optimal patient:* This step is critical. Identify a patient who moved successfully through the continuum offered by your system. Remember, this is an educational vehicle to demonstrate the continuum in action—how the patient progressed from acute care, received services in progressively more independent settings, went home more quickly and more independently, and has demonstrated a good outcome. As mentioned previously, this is extremely important in oncology, because many persons do not recognize the benefit of continuum services after cancer or cancer treatment.

Provider Name
Case Study No. 1:

Provider Name
Address
City, State Zip Code
Phone Number

Insert facility map here

Directions:
(Add directions here)

This case study was prepared and distributed to health care professionals as a community education service.

(Add provider continuum services listing or other information here.)

Patient:
XX year old
Diagnoses on Acute Care
Admission:
-
-
-
-

Medical History:
-

Date of Onset:
X-XX-9X

Date of Specialty Program:
Y-YY-9Y

Reason for Hospital Admission:
-

Social History:
-

Identified Problems and
Barriers to Overcome:
-
-
-

Treatment Plan:
ST: ZZ weeks/X treatment per week
-

PT: Y weeks/Z treatments per day
-

OT: X weeks/Z treatments per week
-

- Nursing Daily

RT: Y days/Z treatments per day
-

Discharge Outcome:
-

Discharge Status:
-
-

2. *Choose good sources:* Talk to nurses on the specialty floors, surgical, oncology, rehab, and so on. Determine if they all mention several of the same patients as you explain your need to identify appropriate candidates. Traditionally, these patients tug on our heartstrings; everyone has favorites and remembers them fondly, because of their family, condition, or courage. These patients touch our lives. Ask several physicians. Start with the oncologist, radiation oncologist, or physiatrist.

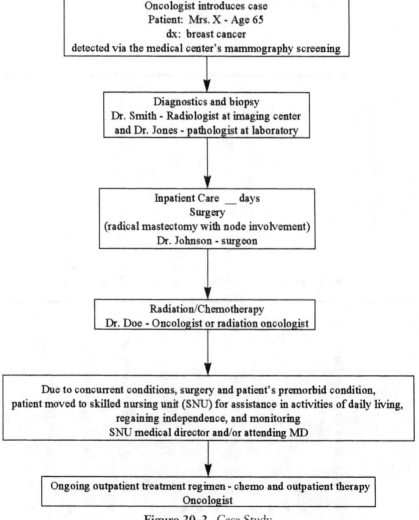

Figure 20–2. Case Study

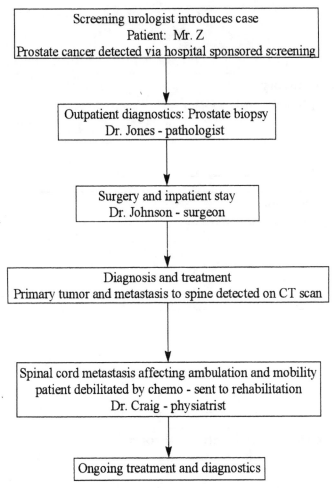

Figure 20–3. Case Study

3. *Qualify your choice:* Check the charts of the selected patients to confirm that they did indeed move successfully through the continuum with a good outcome. Construct a preliminary flowchart for each of them including steps in the process, physicians, and length of stays on each unit (see Figures 20–2 and 20–3 for samples, and Figure 20–4 for a blank worksheet).

4. *Make the final selection of patients:* Now is the time to approach the medical director of the oncology program or the section chief and

Case Study—Diabetes
Mrs. A

Patient History:
Mrs. A presented with . . .

Treatment Goals:
The goals for Mrs. A were . . .

Barriers to Success:
Because of Mrs. A's . . .

Interventions and Treatment Progress:
As she began treatment and education sessions, Mrs. A . . .

Outcomes and Ongoing Issues:

Figure 20–4

present this project. Obtain approval and have the director select one of the suggested patients. If he or she is extremely involved, it may be advisable to approach the other physicians involved and coordinate a team approach with the medical staff office or the education department. As always, be available to assist in whatever way facilitates the project's completion.

5. *Coordinate with the medical staff or education department:* Do this so that they know the educational event is scheduled and promoted. Not always, but often, such an event will all be handled through these avenues and will require little of your assistance (see our sample promotional flyer, Figure 20–5). Will you include hospital-based employees (nurses, therapists, and technicians) in the invitation to the event? (This may not be the best approach; if not, set up a second performance to follow in a timely fashion. You are arranging the event so that physicians will have to prepare only once. Be considerate to their time constraints.

Will you include internal and external referral sources to the continuum in the invitation, such as the facility's social services/discharge planning, utilization review, or case-management professions across the continuum services? This is appropriate when your facility offers a service that fills a niche in a network. You may consider inviting other facilities' professionals who refer to your continuum service and offer the program over breakfast or lunch. Social workers and discharge planners from other facilities may be more likely to attend if the event is a breakfast event on the way to work. In this scenario, they do not actually report to and then leave the facility. As we all know, the logistics of getting away from our offices and our facility can be a challenge, to say the least. Make a few phone calls and determine if a breakfast or luncheon is best. Many organizations shy away from events after working hours or late in the day when attendance may be diminished.

6. The Timing: Because a luncheon presentation by its nature is time limited, make the total presentation time approximately 50 minutes. This allows attendees to get lunch and settle in. Starting promptly is important, since physicians and other medical staff are busy and every department is on a tight personnel budget. Be considerate of your medical staff, employees, and patients. Allocating time to presenters may be the biggest challenge. Explain that you have limited presentation time to accommodate staff schedules.

Grand Rounds:
The Continuum of Care—Cancer

Monday, November 3

The Chilton Room   Noon to 1 P.M.
Lunch begins
at 11:45

Mrs. X, Breast Cancer Patient

Presented by

Dr. Joe Smith, oncologist

Dr. Tyler Crain, radiologist

Dr. Lee Brown, surgeon

Dr. Ken Lee, pathologist

Dr. Bryce Arnold, radiation oncologist

Dr. Gary Glaser, physiatrist

Figure 20–5

FAMILY REFERENCE NETWORK SHEETS

The format: An 8½-by-11-inch sheet on facility or program letterhead, typeface same as facility identity.

The project: A listing of your references, family members, or former patients who will vouch for your program and its outcomes.

The method: Approach a number of former patients and family members who were pleased with your program and who had excellent outcomes. Develop the lists by diagnosis if your program serves more than one focus or condition. Phone the individuals and ask if they would agree to participate in this program. Sometimes people are very pleased to do this; in other cases, it is not convenient. Explain to them that this list will be used in the final stage of decision making with families, and will not be just given out to every caller. Honor their wishes. List times at which someone could phone; no one wants calls at all hours. Do not list addresses, just names. You may wish to give only first names and phone numbers.

Network sheets can be effective tools and can help establish a support system for families who often need such an avenue. Some program directors and administrators of skilled and assisted living facilities prefer to conduct this activity more informally. At the end of tours they introduce the prospect to a family member or resident who has agreed to participate in a private conversation regarding the facility or program.

Medicare Part B Brochures (For Long-Term Care or Assisted Living)

Format: Use a small double sided trifold brochure on an 8½-by-11-inch sheet of paper or preprinted shell; typeface and colors should be consistent with those of the system or facility.

Goal: To promote Medicare Part B ancillary services to those individuals who may benefit from them because of their decline in function or potential for increased independence (see our sample trifold in Figure 20–6).

Brief, concise descriptions of services offered:

- *OT—Occupational Therapy:* This can be very helpful in increasing independence in the activities of daily living, such as bathing, dressing, and grooming. Adaptive devices may be available to facilitate the pride and dignity of self-capability.

MAINTAINING INDEPENDENCE AT ANY AGE

After therapy services have maximized an individual's capabilities and no further gains can be made, Medicare regulations require the transition of this care to another department of the nursing facility, so that it is fully covered within the costs of the facility. There is no additional cost. This function is called restorative care and the goal of this function is to maintain the advances made in therapy. The facility will have at least one individual who is a restorative aide, focusing on patients who need assistance in maintaining their level of independence. Nursing facilities can offer increased levels of independence to many patients through therapy services and the opportunity to maintain a level of independence through the facility's restorative nursing program.

Ask the Rehabilitation Program Manager or the facility's Social Worker to tell you more about how therapy may assist someone you love in becoming more independent.

Figure 20–6

Whether we are 5 or 95, our feelings is the same—"I'd rather do it myself." We smile fondly at children who struggle into their clothes, want to perform bathing and grooming tasks alone and say, "Don't help me!," but now as adults we may take this level of independence for granted.

When we admit a parent or loved one to an assisted living or nursing facility, we suddenly expect that the individual will simply acquiesce to being done for and accept the situation. We forget that not so long ago when they were at home or within our home, they took pride in their independence, no matter what the task.

Daily care and activities at any nursing facility are an important aspect of the care of an individual, but the hope of reaching and maintaining some levels of independence are paramount to the individual's quality of life. This is recognized by Medicare and reimbursement for this care is provided through Medicare Part B, which you may be familiar with as it covers physicians' visits.

Medicare Part B generally covers Physical Therapy, Occupational Therapy, and Speech Therapy, if it is medically necessary and ordered by a physician. Part B Medicare reimbursement is generally at 80%, just as in physician office visits and a supplemental insurance policy may cover the remainder. If there is no supplemental policy, the patient or family is responsible for the remaining cost for the short term therapy.

Physical Therapy- The goal is to move the patient toward greater independent mobility either unassisted or with assistive devices. The licensed physical therapists focus on improving coordination, balance, strength and endurance.

Occupational Therapy- The goal is to assess personal self care and daily living skills providing modified techniques and/or adaptive devices as necessary to assist the patient to adapt their capabilities to skills needed in the activities of daily living.

Speech Therapy- The goal is to address communication problems by helping patients improve skills in speaking, listening, thinking, reading, writing, problem solving and sequencing thoughts. The therapist may also assess swallowing difficulties and develop treatment and management programs to address the patient's condition.

- *PT—Physical Therapy:* This can be helpful for people experiencing decreased mobility. Physical therapists can offer gait training, as well as instruction on the use of canes, walkers, and wheelchairs.

- *SLP—Speech Language Pathologists:* Speech therapy addresses both cognitive deficits and ways to improve communication, both verbal and written. In addition, speech therapists work with people experiencing dysphagia (difficulty swallowing), a serious problem that can lead to life-threatening complications.

- *Restorative Care:* Restorative care is offered to help people maintain gains made as a result of therapy. In skilled facilities, restorative care is part of routine care and is generally performed by a certified nurse's aide who has received training through the therapy department.

- *Financials:* Discuss the particulars of Medicare outpatient coverage and supplemental policies so that coverage is understood. There are several free governmental publications regarding Medicare available through the Health Care Financing Administration.

BROWN BAG LUNCHEON SERIES

Members of the healthcare community may benefit from a monthly brown bag luncheon series. This is an informal lecture/networking series offering no continuing education units (CEUs). By not offering CEUs, the group can be kept to a manageable size. This gives focus to learning informally about different continuum components rather than getting required CEUs. Of course, CEUs are an option if indicated in your community, or if you have sufficient room to manage the groups attending and a staff member or department who can process the CEU requests with state organizations.

Begin by developing a list of approximately fifty persons who could benefit from education regarding the provider's services. Physicians, their office staffs, social workers and discharge planning professionals, nursing facility administrators, and home health representatives may be included. Next, look for topics that are both educational and promotional in their nature. Then schedule the luncheons. Limit attendance according to the space available.

Your dietary department can make the brown bag lunches and receive credit via "Compliments of Provider" stickers. Order napkins in the provider's color with its logo. These small touches make everything more special and are good marketing. Use them when you take box luncheons out to physician offices, as well. This is a good vehicle for meeting key people and developing relationships that will be beneficial.

At first you may want to offer a small honorarium to speakers. Generally, however, they are glad to present without compensation. Expert speakers may include program directors, physicians, and representatives from Medicare and Medicaid. Eventually, attendees will suggest speakers. Focus on retaining the quality of the presentations and on balancing the marketing of the provider's continuum services with information about outside experts and community services. Local specialty hospitals may also present. Other providers with complementary services may share their expertise for the benefit of patients.

EDUCATIONAL SEMINARS

Physicians also may go on the road to promote their services to outlying senior centers. One marketing director presented a four-week summer program that featured staff physicians presenting on such topics as heat stroke, keeping your mind fit in the summer, skin cancer, and summer nutrition. Presentations were conducted by an internist, a psychiatrist, a plastic surgeon, and a registered dietitian.

Presentations to the public can be highly successful. Years ago when I worked as a marketing director in Melborne, Fla., I approached the American Cancer Society (ACS) to cosponsor a program on food choices and healthy dining out. At that time they offered a complete program, ad, logo, and brochures on this subject. I met with the chef at the most desirable hotel in our beachfront community (part of a large national chain) and enlisted him to speak on choosing healthy meals when dining out. Everyone enjoyed the presentation, and it was well attended. The ACS provided their logo for the advertisement and a local radio station picked up the public service announcements at no charge.

JOINT REPLACEMENT SEMINAR OUTLINE AND CHECKLIST

This is a presentation to educate about joint replacements. Each seminar features a different orthopedic surgeon or group to conduct a relatively short presentation on indications for joint replacement, the actual procedure, and the continuum of care for these patients. Components include:

- Handouts/brochures
- Videotape excerpts from surgery
- A representative from the vendor that provides the types of joints used in surgery, with a table set up so that people can see and feel the artificial joints
- At least one patient from the physician's practice who has had surgery and has experienced the continuum at your hospital. The physician generally introduces the patient, who tells about his or her experience.
- Refreshments
- Name tags and a sign-in sheet to secure a mailing list

I coordinated one of these seminars in a town on the Central Florida Coast. The main speaker, an orthopedic surgeon, had a large practice and was a strong supporter of rehabilitation. We placed one Sunday print ad and used broadcast public-service spots for promotion. We had more than 100 attendees. We enlisted a vendor who displayed an array of joint replacement hardware. Attendees liked seeing and holding the hardware, and they marveled over the technology that had changed the other patients' lives. They enjoyed the opportunity to listen to peers who had undergone the joint replacement. All of the physicians' patients who attended wore shorts and skirts and "modeled" their surgical scars (in the knee area) and new smooth gait for the audience. We were later able to track patients back to this event.

STAGING THE EVENT

Approximately Ninety Days to One Month Out:

- Target orthopedic surgeon; obtain date(s) of availability
- Establish day, date, and time; evening or afternoon, day of the week, depending on the demographics and preferences of the senior population in your local area, time of year (darkness factor), and room availability
- Reserve room

- Confirm with physician; request the name of the vendor representative who supplies the hardware for the operations; request permission to secure the rep's assistance through the physician's referral
- Ask the physician if he or she would like to invite a "success case" patient from the practice to participate. Determine how you can help to facilitate this; usually the physicians have good relationships with these patients and the patients are flattered to be asked to participate and relate their experience.
- Phone the vendor representatives for participation. They may or may not offer to cover the costs of refreshments as an exhibitor courtesy. Handle this according to the policy of your organization.
- Submit catering request to your dietary department
- Reserve audiovisual equipment as needed. This is an older audience; you may need several VCRs so that everyone can see. If you will be selecting the video consider it well: from different vantage points, blood-and-gore ratings, and so on. While television programs have long been set in medical, surgical, and ER settings, this may be disconcerting to some people. A good screening tool is to ask someone you know who has no medical background to watch the tape. If the physician will be making this choice from his or her library, introduce these considerations and offer to assist in screening the tape.
- Finalize marketing strategy and budget; print and broadcast advertising, direct mail, flyers in physician's office, and so on. Determine if you will specify that "This event is free, but seating is limited. Please phone to reserve your seats." This may alleviate seating and refreshment shortages. Take the ad to the physician for approval. Offer copies of the ad for the physician's office. Finally, place ads.

Two Weeks Before Event

- Reconfirm with physician and confirm patient participation.
- Determine if the practice has any brochures to make available on the sign-in table, request brochures from your own provider or continuum programs.

One Week Before Event

- Pick up brochures from physician's office. Chat with office staff about the event.
- Double-check all arrangements.
- Double-check patient "success case" participation, transportation to event, and so on.
- Determine if ads have run, or are running.
- Begin daily monitoring of responses—RSVPs.
- Assemble packets or brochures from physician office and your provider.

Day of Event

- Check responses against arrangements, check weather conditions, and so on.
- Check in with physician; advise him or her on prospective size of group and other pertinent details.
- Arrive early to set up room; set out packets, name tags, and sign-in sheet; check arrangements; assist physician; check A/V equipment, adjust lighting; check room temperature, and post directional signs at all doors.

After the Event

- Send thank-you notes to those who helped staff the event, including the physician and vendor rep.
- Have all names and addresses entered into a database. Provide a list to the physician's office and your provider's admissions staff for their tracking purposes, matching new patients in the practice to the event attendance list. Send thank you or follow-up mailing to attendees, and maintain the list for future direct-mail and tracking purposes.

ARTHRITIS AND HAND SCREENINGS

Depending upon the depth of your continuum and the focus of physicians, arthritis screenings are excellent marketing and screening tools for the health of the community. We offer this schedule to hold a screening in your area in concert with members of your medical staff.

STAGING THE EVENT
Approximately Ninety Days Out:

- Meet with physicians. You may conduct the screening with one physician or you may offer the service to all orthopedists on staff.
- Set date and time of screening. Allow for appointments to be booked all day or for half a day. Determine staff required, that is, physical therapy (PT), occupational therapy (OT), and support staff. While patients are waiting for their appointment or after their appointment, an OT can give paraffin hand baths or conduct demonstrations on assistive devices that can make activities of daily living (bathing, grooming, and dressing) easier. A PT can talk about energy conservation and posture and demonstrate therapeutic exercise. A home health or program nurse can use charts and pictures to illustrate the different types of arthritis, charts showing carpal tunnel syndrome, and so on, and how these disorders affect the body. Office staff can help the doctor's staff in registering attendees and showing them to an exam room, marketing the physician's practice as they do so.
- Discuss the potential value with physician(s), particularly the opportunity to increase their patient base and provide a service to the community.
- Discuss marketing budget, including the advertising budget, collaterals, any specialty items to be given away, and refreshments.
- Begin working on marketing collaterals, if needed, including working with a writer/designer, contacting the Arthritis Foundation for pamphlets, and ordering pamphlets from different organizations, such as the American Academy of Orthopedic Surgeons, for different diagnoses, and pamphlets showing such techniques as joint replacement surgery.
- Decide who will be responsible for scheduling appointments. If only one physician is involved, it's easier for his or her

office to book appointments. If multiple physicians are involved, it's easier and more appropriate to develop a centralized scheduling process out of the marketing department.
- Arrange for staff and set their schedules.

Approximately Sixty Days Out:

- Write ads and press releases announcing the event.
- Contact vendors about refreshments and displays with artificial joints.

Approximately Thirty Days Out

- Contact all media in your service area. Try to go in person, if possible, for the smaller papers. Invite the media to the event.
- Buy ad space
- Suggest a story on physician(s) and the disease to be screened (arthritis).

Last Month Before Screening:

- Contact physician's office weekly to track the number of appointments scheduled.
- Confirm details, such as paraffin bath demos, therapy demos, equipment demos (activities of daily living assistive devices); finalize staff details, such as who will be giving tours, and welcoming and registering patients.
- Follow-Up Notes: After the screening, follow up with the doctor's office staff on an ongoing basis to keep track of the numbers and names of new patients they received from the screening. Enter the names of all attendees into the database for orthopedic marketing. Send thank-you notes to those who staffed the event. A short follow-up story to newspapers may be appropriate.

PHYSICIANS' OFFICE PATIENT SIGN-IN SHEETS

On a recent trip to central Florida we called on physicians' offices. Several office staff members told us that the level of marketing in the area was intense, with four to five marketers calling on the offices daily. They noted that four out of five were from home health agencies. While standing at the window we couldn't help noticing the pads of sign-in sheets for patients at the windows of several offices. The traditional sign-in pads with numbers and lines for patients to sign in had commercials on the bottom of the sheet. We were able to review sheets for two home health providers and one subacute nursing facility.

This is a very effective promotional tool, conveying the message to the exact target market in a very subtle way. Physicians' offices will no doubt accept pads for sign-in that they would otherwise have to print on their own. Marketers have a reason to drop by periodically and have props that speak for them all day long. Individuals visiting their physician may one day need the service or know someone who will. They are more likely to have name recognition when the referral is made. We give this idea an "A."

PUBLIC EDUCATION—ARTHRITIS

Public education is a great service to our community. It is especially useful in the case of arthritis, so that treatment may begin early to decrease the progression as much as possible. The Arthritis Foundation is involved with education programs and many other services for the benefit of those with the condition. You may contact the local chapter to determine the actual extent of services. According to their publication *Arthritis: Do You Know?* services may include educational programs, exercise classes, self-care classes, and support groups. Although you may develop you own materials, we include the following suggestions:

ARTHRITIS EDUCATION PROGRAM (OVERHEADS OR SLIDES)

The goal is to increase the attendees' knowledge of arthritis and services offered by the healthcare organization for those with the condition.

- Visual No. 1—The introduction includes a brief overview of the presentation and why the individual leading the seminar is qualified to do so. It briefly mentions only the continuum services available.
- Visual Nos. 2 and 3—Definitions and descriptions are presented, with visuals of normal and affected joints and causes.

- Visual No. 4—Children and adults can develop arthritis.
- Visuals—Different types of arthritis.
- Visuals—Treatment of arthritis to include diagnostics, medications, surgical interventions, use of modalities (heat and cold), joint protection, energy conservation techniques, and other self-help techniques.
- Visuals—Misconceptions and unproven remedies (refer to the booklet of the same name by the Arthritis Foundation).
- Visuals—Warning signs of arthritis.
- Visuals—Arthritis services and resources within the community and the healthcare organization continuum.
- Summary and closing comments.

PUBLIC EDUCATION—DIABETES

Diabetes education is a tremendous service for the public because many who may have the disease have not been diagnosed. We are providing the service for the health of our community. (See Figures 20–7 and 20–8 for sample announcements for diabetes education programs.) In the past, marketers conducted community education as a soft sell to attract patients into the system. While today it is still somewhat of a soft sell for the continuum as a whole, we are trying also to alleviate acute care admissions for the benefit of the patient, the payor, and the healthcare system. Keep in mind that many consultants would assert that 35 percent of the inpatient days from Medicare risk contract patients can be ICU days. No matter how focused hospitals are on reducing length of stay, we can only shave days off the back end of an inpatient stay—not the front end of the admission. The most costly financial implication of the admission is at the front of the stay, and the only potential to manage costs will be by keeping the patients healthier and out of the hospital.

PUBLIC EDUCATION—STROKE

Potential topics in stroke education are numerous, as are the resources available. The National Stroke Association and the American Heart Association produce excellent educational materials. Additional materials are no doubt available from many other associations and companies. The Internet is also a valuable resource. Courses may be developed through in-house options (continuing education departments or individual programs) or may be externally purchased. Appropriate topics in this area abound, including warning signs of stroke, understanding stroke, and life after a stroke. Many facilities offer blood-pressure screenings as a service to the community as part of their cardiac or neurology programs.

Sample Outline for Stroke Education

Format: Hand out packet on facility letterhead with complimentary booklets for the families and attendees from resources as suggested above.

Visuals: Slides, overheads, or brief videos (C. Everett Koop hosts on a set available through retail outlets) are a nice addition to mix delivery vehicles. (Keep in mind that some individuals are visual and some are auditory in their learning styles, so mix the delivery for maximum effectiveness). Many computer software and CD-ROM programs offer medical illustrations and have detailed anatomy of the brain. This type of illustration is well suited to the lay audience.

- Visual No. 1—This is the introduction to the presentation and to what you hope to impart to the audience. It is the overview of what will be addressed.
- Visual No. 2—For marketing impact this should include a brief discussion of the services provided by your facility or system, as well as an explanation of why your facility is qualified to educate in this area. The speaker's credentials also should be introduced here.
- Visual No. 3—A visual of the normal brain. Explain how the brain works, and how it is nourished by an extensive blood supply.
- Visual No. 4—Discuss the different regions of the brain and the function of the body that each controls, such as language, movement, and balance. (Include an explanation of right-brain damage versus left-brain damage.) An excellent resource is the booklet *How Stroke Affects Behavior* from the American Heart Association.

THE DIABETES MANAGEMENT SERIES

OUTPATIENT TEACHING PROGRAM

SPONSORED BY

THE PROVIDER NAME
ADDRESS

Presented by our certified diabetes educators

"THE DIABETES DIAGNOSIS"

featuring

**What you need to know on:
Diabetes
Medications
Preventing complications
Managing your diet and exercise
Controlling your response
Taking responsibility for your lifestyle**

Saturday, January 14

8 A.M. to noon

*The cost of this outpatient teaching program is $ _____ .
Please phone 000-0000 to reserve your seat.*

Figure 20–7

FREE COMMUNITY EDUCATION PROGRAM

"DIABETES UPDATE"

An update on the most current treatments and advances
in the treatment of diabetes

featuring: Dr. Tyler Keaton

Tuesday, February 11
7 P.M. to 8 P.M.

in
THE HERITAGE ROOM

THE PROVIDER NAME
ADDRESS

*This seminar is free, but seating is limited.
Please phone to reserve your seat(s).*

Figure 20–8

- Visual No. 5—The brain, with an illustration of a disruption in the blood supply. Discuss what happens when the stroke occurs in different areas and how the stroke can extend after it has initially occurred. Again, the American Heart Association offers a booklet, *Strokes: A Guide for the Family*, which has an excellent discussion of how strokes occur. Discuss the types of stroke and causes.

- Visual No. 6—Treatment of a stroke. This discussion outlines the immediate care for a person with stroke—diagnosis, treatment, and progression through the provider's continuum of care to skilled care, rehabilitation (outpatient and inpatient), or home health care.

- Visuals No. 7 and on—Some providers will insert more detailed information about their continuum at this point and add visuals.

- Visual—Life after stroke. People have misconceptions regarding recovery after a stroke, such as capabilities and sex after stroke. This is a general discussion with the recognition of the different levels of stroke and the residual effects. Again, the American Heart Association's booklet *How Stroke Affects Behavior* presents a good explanation of many considerations in interacting with a stroke survivor.

- Visual—List and discuss the risk factors of stroke such as atherosclerosis and high blood pressure. Discuss the value of working with one's physician to take responsibility for one's own health and attempting to minimize risk factors as much as possible.

- Visual—Recognizing a stroke. Unfortunately, many people do not know that immediate recognition of the warning signs of stroke and early intervention can affect the course of a stroke. Refer to the American Heart Association's publication, *Heart Attack and Stroke: Signals and Action* for an excellent overview of the warning signs and the need for immediate response.

- Final Visual—Summarize and close with a discussion of your services and the provider's commitment to the community in providing education services.

SUPPORT GROUPS

Individuals, family members, and caregivers can often receive tremendous benefit from participation in support groups, no matter what the diagnosis. The support group concept is applicable to many illnesses and conditions that affect individuals' daily lives. Support groups serve several different functions:

- Education—Unfortunately, with the shortening of acute care lengths of stay and the shifting of hospitals to providers for acute episodes, patients and their caregivers have less opportunity for education with knowledgeable professionals. These groups generally provide guest speakers, books, articles, and other information useful in providing an understanding of the disease process.
- Community resource connections—Support groups can often link members and those inquiring with community resources.
- Support—Facing such life changes can sometimes be easier if they are not faced alone. The support of others who are facing or who have faced the challenges and are willing to share their experiences can be invaluable.

Many hospitals and organizations sponsor support groups as a public service. Other facilities that do not have sufficient resources to undertake sole sponsorship of a group will often provide meeting space and refreshments to such groups. Cooperation between providers is also key within a community. We have seen two major providers of postacute services within the same community jointly sponsor a group and alternate the setting monthly. Providers can pool resources so that individual organization commitments are lessened. Many organizations sponsor support groups and can make available a listing of those in local areas.

ELECTIVE ORTHOPEDIC SURGERY CONTINUUM PREADMISSION PROGRAMS

As the population of the United States grows older, the incidence of elective joint procedures is expected to rise. Given the nature of elective surgery, hospitals have the opportunity to promote the continuum

CONTINUUM FLOW CHART FOR ORTHOPEDIC ADMISSION

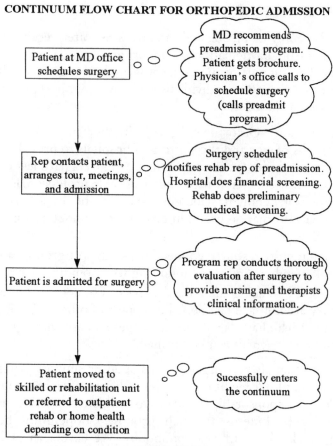

Figure 20–9

of care services before actual admission to the hospital. This is an opportunity to manage the expectations of the public, the patient, and referral sources through both promotional campaigns and one-to-one education.

The preadmission program is a systems process within a facility. A successful approach will require a dedication of personnel resources to facilitate the process. Many organizations are attempting to increase their market share and revenues by attracting more patients with little focus on moving the patients they have through the system in a cost-effective method. The preadmission approach to orthopedic patients has the potential to decrease slippage from the system and to attract new patients through marketing the continuum of care (refer to Figure 20–9).

Mechanism

- Patients scheduled for elective orthopedic surgery (primarily hip and knee procedures) are "preadmitted" for inpatient or outpatient rehabilitation or home health services when identified by their physician.
- While the patient is in the physician's office, the physician or office staff gives the patient an orthopedic continuum of care brochure and explains that patients often benefit from these services in their recovery and pursuit of greater independence.
- Supply brochures with holders to the physician offices.
- Hospital gets the patient's name and number via surgical scheduling. (Obviously this will take some coordination as the system is implemented.)
- The continuum representative phones the patient to schedule rehabilitation, manage expectations; offer to meet with patient and family if necessary, and provide a "what to bring" list and map or explanation of outpatient/home health care.
- Upon the patient's admission to the hospital, the admitting clerk discusses the continuum of care, offers a brochure, and responds to the patient's expectations.
- Unit personnel and case management reinforce the continuum of care through the stay and discharge planning.
- Continuum of care brochures are in surgical waiting areas and in containers mounted on the backs of patient room doors.
- Patient is referred to and begins continuum services.

Advantages:

- Working through orthopedic surgeons to identify appropriate patients and educate them while managing their expectations.
- Facilitating appropriate patient admissions into the continuum of care services in an efficient and cost-effective manner.

- Managing census and staffing issues with more information regarding prospective admissions.
- Obtaining better preliminary clinical information on patients to plan rehabilitation goals (inpatient, skilled, outpatient, and home health).

Key Points for Success:

- Effective brochure placed in appropriate areas
- Surgeon's complete support
- Coordination between surgical scheduling, physician's office, and continuum manager
- Discharge-planning functions focused on the continuum

DRG FOCUS PROJECTS

Acute care hospitals often use this type of project to educate physicians about their own continuums as they manage the length of stay for problem DRG areas.

The UR or finance department identifies the DRGs that are of concern to the organization. Within the DRG they also identify the average length of stay (ALOS) for the facility and the target ALOS (budgeted, state, national, etc.). Some hospitals have chosen to include the average outlier costs to the hospital by DRG, as well. (Just what to list is at the administration's discretion.)

The individual DRGs with corresponding information are put onto posters, under discretionary information. Some facilities choose to prompt referrals by including several utilization management questions about the condition that would lead to different continuum components. For example, could the individual benefit from skilled services? Can they be sent home with home health? If the skilled unit is new, perhaps the poster could outline the criteria for skilled admission. These posters are tailored to the needs of the facility (identifying DRGs to target) and promoting continuum component usage.

This type of project lends itself to creative license, and does not have to be used in the acute hospital setting exclusively. It would also be helpful to the non-hospital-based organization with extensive services to focus everyone on the most effective utilization.

ORTHOPEDIC CONTINUUM OF CARE BROCHURE CONSIDERATIONS

While your advertising agency will have its own ideas about developing continuum of care brochures, the following are a few ideas and an outline to help you get started and help guard your advertising dollars.

Specifications

- Use matte finish.
- Line graphics rather than photos can save money.
- Type size and font should reflect your current identity.
- Type should accommodate older readers.

Outline

A. Introduction
  1. Acknowledges the plan for surgery
  2. Positions the continuum of care as augmenting, not replacing, the quality care offered by the patient's physician
  3. Focuses on the progressive independence goal to return the patient to home or an alternative care setting
  4. Briefly names the continuum components and includes a continuum graphic

B. Explanation of joint-replacement surgeries and admitting procedures for your hospital
  1. Hip/knee surgery information—A brief, nontechnical description of why and how a joint is repaired or replaced. Use illustrations. (These are available on CD-ROM at computer stores for little cost.)
  2. Admitting procedures—A brief discussion of what to bring (identification, insurance cards, personal items, etc.) and any other pertinent information.

C. Surgical/postsurgical information—This is basic information that a patient might find helpful such as:
  1. Preparations for what to expect before and during surgery while the patient is still in his or her room
  2. Location of the family or surgical waiting area
  3. Recovery room, how long the patient is there, and why

   4. Return to the patient's room
   5. Physician's visits throughout the continuum services
D. The continuum components
   1. One brief paragraph reiterating the goal of progressive
       independence and listing of the continuum services in
       your hospital or system
   2. Once concise paragraph on each of the services you may
       offer
      a. Skilled/subacute
      b. Physical rehabilitation (inpatient or outpatient)
      c. Home health
      d. Long-term care/assisted living
E. Summary points
   1. Your system provides the spectrum of services to focus
       on the goals of increased independence.
   2. The patient's physician is a part of this continuum of care.
   3. Physicians are encouraged to follow patients through the
       continuum of care. Reports will be sent to physicians on
       the patient's progress and discharge.
   4. Even if patients choose to go home and later believe that
       they could benefit from the continuum of care, you may be
       able to assist them in providing the services that they need.

CORONARY CONTINUUM OF CARE BROCHURE CONSIDERATIONS

Many progressive facilities have been promoting their cardiac continuum as a package for years. But they have not always included all facets
of the continuum, such as skilled or home health care, in addition to
the cardiac rehab services and diagnostics. The following is a sample
outline to start your creative juices flowing.

Specifications

- Use low gloss or matte finish paper.
- Use graphics or photos (consider black-and-white art to save
  money).
- Type size and font should reflect the facility's current identity
  and support.
- Should be clear and readable.

Outline

A. Introduction
   1. Acknowledges cardiac condition
   2. Positions the continuum of care as augmenting, not replacing, the quality care offered by the patient's physician
   3. Focuses on the progressive independence goal and return to home, work, and the community
   4. Briefly names the continuum components and includes a continuum graphic

B. Brief introduction to cardiac conditions; maintain an educational focus in layman's terms

C. Critical-care stage—An explanation of the critical-care stage may include brief comments regarding the ER, ICU, and coronary care unit (CCU). This includes the high-tech focus on coronary care and the personal care provided by specially trained physicians and nurses.

   This section should also include practical information such as the visitation policy for ICU and CCU and the rationale for this (what it means for patients). Also cover personal belongings and get-well gifts. (Because of the heart monitoring equipment in every room, space for get-well gifts is limited. Perhaps they should be held until after the patient is ready to leave the CCU.)

D. Initial recovery/progressive recovery—An explanation of the first step after leaving the critical stage. This may include cardiac step-down, skilled/subacute, cardiac monitoring, discharge from the hospital with inpatient/outpatient cardiac rehab, home health, etc.

E. Outpatient cardiac rehab—This section continues the concept of progressive recovery and discusses the twelve-week, thirty-six-session progressive program. The focus of this section is that this program is designed for those who want to take more responsibility for the management of their cardiac condition. It stresses the educational and monitored exercise components.

   This section also addresses the eligibility requirements for Medicare and the importance of completing the course, given the Medicare limit on sessions.

Also addressed is insurance reimbursement. For example, some insurance companies have set their own requirements for coverage. The hospital will work with the patient to determine the coverage available through insurance.

F. Maintaining a healthy approach to your cardiac condition— This section discusses ongoing educational programs offered by the hospital and continuing under a physician's care. The point of this section is an educational focus on management of the cardiac condition.

G. Summary points

1. Your hospital/network provides the spectrum of services (technology and medical professionals) to focus on the cardiac continuum of care.

2. The patient's physician is part of this continuum of care.

3. There are advantages in staying within the continuum of care.

4. Physicians are encouraged to follow patients through the continuum of care. Reports will be sent to physicians regarding patient progress throughout the continuum.

5. Even if patients go home and later believe that they could benefit from cardiac rehabilitation, you may be able to assist them in providing the services that they need.

RESOURCES

The following is a listing of organizations that may be helpful to you in your marketing efforts.

- American Academy of Orthopaedic Surgeons
  6300 N. River Road
  Rosemont, IL 60018
- American Cancer Association
  1599 Clifton Road NE
  Atlanta, GA 30329-4251
- American Heart Association
  7272 Greenville Ave.
  Dallas, TX 72231-4596
- American Diabetes Association
  1660 Duke St.
  Alexandria, VA 22314

- Arthritis Foundation
  P.O. Box 19000
  Atlanta, GA 30326
- Alzheimer's Disease and Related Disorders Association
  919 N. Michigan Ave.
  Chicago, IL 60611-1676

SUMMARY

We encourage the reader to consider the samples included within this chapter and to creatively tailor them to individual components across the continuum. Resources listed in this chapter and in Chapter 1 are available, and they can be of value in the education and marketing process. We will look forward to seeing your ideas during our mystery shopping across the nation.

21

CHAPTER

Implementation and Management of the Direct Education Contact Effort

While specialty programs have long used the one-to-one direct education contact (sales call) as the core of their marketing efforts, a few rotten apples have spoiled the concept for many in healthcare. Please keep in mind that this effort may be conducted appropriately, effectively, and *ethically*. The issue beginning to arise now is not so much how to conduct the effort but how to pull it all together when there is an entire continuum to promote and multiple representatives all identifying and calling upon some of the same potential targets. (This is surely the quickest way to alienate the medical staff!). An added complication for many hospitals is the presence of vendors or management companies who operate and market the specialty units and programs.

Hospital-based managers will become increasingly responsible for managing the promotional efforts of their units and programs, and in some facilities this is creating new challenges and opportunities. In this chapter, we will provide an overview of:

- Identifying referral sources
- Tips on selecting the right representative
- Cross-training

- Contact planning and rotation schedules
- Evaluating and monitoring the effort

Marketing techniques are those historically used to promote specialty services, including:

- Identifying referral sources to target
- Development of the approach to each market segment
- Conducting the one-to-one contact and maintaining communication
- Monitoring success of the effort and redefining the referral sources to target

IDENTIFYING REFERRAL SOURCES

Referral sources are segmented into:

- Immediate census builders: Those individuals who have patients immediately to be referred to specialty services. These are generally hospital based, such as staff nurses, therapists, and social workers/discharge planners/case managers/utilization review/utilization management
- Intermediate census builders: Those individuals who may not have patients today but who will likely have them in the near future, such as physicians
- Longer-term census builders: Those individuals who will eventually come into contact with others who may require specialty services, such as insurance case managers and members of community groups, support groups, clergy, or the public

Approach to Immediate Census Builders

Their Need	Your Focus
Providers who will meet their needs, moving patients in a timely fashion.	The efficiency of your admissions system.
Providers who can meet the educational needs of prospective patients, freeing up the immediate census builder to move to the next patient.	Ability to meet with patient, family or decision maker, arrange tours, explain financial coverage, etc.

Providers who will not be nuisances constantly marketing to them.

Your readiness and ability to respond; with periodic phone calls and less-frequent visits than other marketers "trolling" the halls.

On-Site Preadmission Assessments

- Assist in patient/family education during discharge-planning process.
- Family and patient interaction during on-site assessment.
- Provision of program-specific materials, such as a packet of information and biography sheets on direct care providers.

Other Amenities

- Arrange tours and transport the family to facility for tour if necessary.
- Provision of: *Your Medicare Handbook 199X.*
  The facility may order these free from the U.S. Department of Health and Human Services at:

  Health Care Financing Administration
  6325 Security Boulevard
  Baltimore, Maryland 21207-5187
  Publication No. HCFA 10050.

Immediate census builders have the ability to refer patients on any given day, so they should be contacted at least once a week. Phone calls to them are acceptable, as are faxes.

Approach to Intermediate Census Builders

Their Need

A facility that will deliver quality care and meet the demands of patients and families.

A facility they can rely on to facilitate admissions smoothly and quickly.

Your Focus

Promoting the program, and the appropriateness of the setting in delivering quality care.

The ease of the admit process.

A facility that works well with families and receives few complaints.	Working closely with families.
Knowledge of how to bill for visits.	Explaining visits and billing to the physicians who choose to follow patients.
May prefer to have another physician follow patient or to turn over to medical director.	Introducing the physicians who are willing to follow patients.
Need for progress information and return of the patient to the physician's practice.	Explaining the communication procedures with physicians who refer patients, and the return to the practice mechanism that has been established. Most often this may be scheduling the first return appointment with the physician and mailing reports from team conferences during the stay.

Intermediate census builders will eventually have a patient to refer, and then will have more to refer. They should be visited once a month. The optimal way to achieve a relationship with this group is to develop a communication system for admission/discharge notification, reports, and scheduling of a follow-up appointment on discharge. By using this type of approach, the visits will occur more frequently, but will be with a clear purpose. Frequently the contact will be with the office staff, who will convey information to the physician.

Approach to Longer-Term Census Builders

Their Need	**Your Focus**
Efficient admissions process.	No-glitch admissions systems.
Cost of an acute bed vs. a specialty program for the delivery of quality care (insurers).	Costs.

Timely and accurate information.	Reporting and communications systems with referral sources.
The designation of liaison(s) with insurers or external case managers (insurers).	Contact person(s) for questions and communications.
Return of the patient to the referring system.	Return patient mechanism.
Quality delivery of care for appropriate candidates.	Provide quality care in a specialty program setting.

Longer-term census builders will take a longer period of time to build referral patterns. Consider visiting them once a month at first, and then later assess this time line so that you may adjust it in relation to their patient volume. Augment the monthly schedule with phone calls to keep name recognition and visibility high.

CENSUS DEVELOPMENT CONTACT STRATEGY

What is a one-to-one contact? It is a casual or planned meeting: at the hospital, office, or facility (virtually anywhere) with a discussion regarding how to refer, a follow-up on a referral, or introduction of services.

They do the talking. (Remember the 80/20 rule: spend 80 percent of your time listening, 20 percent of your time answering their questions and asking/clarifying points.) Specifically, you should concentrate on the following:

- Briefly explain how the facility or program can meet their expressed needs.
- Gather information regarding their referral patterns or physician practice.
- Qualify and quantify the referral source (how many patients and what type could they refer, to indicate how much time you should dedicate to their referral development).
- Ask for a referral.
- Get the names of other referral contacts.

Success Steps During a Contact and Referral Relationship

- Focus on their needs, knowledge level, and questions. Remember: Ask, don't tell.
- Position yourself as a clinical problem solver who is interested in helping their patients.
- Become actively involved in their referral process and earn their respect by offering accurate information, timely admissions, and follow-up information.

Sample Checklist for Selecting a Representative

- Does he or she have credibility and commitment? A clinician or someone with personal experience within their specialty program area has credibility.
- Is this person a basically friendly, outgoing person? Would you want to talk to this person if you just met them?
- Does this person have a professional appearance and presentation? This person *is* your program.
- Is he or she a highly motivated individual capable of working autonomously? There is potential for a suboptimal performance to be undetected for an extended period of time.
- Can he or she communicate good news and bad news equally effectively to all internal and external markets?
- Is he or she someone who does not resent being referred to as "the one who does sales?"

And the most important consideration is: If the patient was your grandparent or parent, would you refer to this individual? If you must compromise, do so in favor of enthusiasm and belief in the product. Select the candidate that the interview team enjoyed speaking with the most. The perfect candidate may be nonexistent, in light of the wish list above, but it is easier to sell when there is a passion and belief in the product.

CROSS TRAINING THE TEAM TO THINK CONTINUUM AND INTEGRATED DELIVERY SYSTEM

As outlined earlier in the target sheets, hospital employees simply must be educated in the continuum of care provided by the hospital and system. With unit staff and employees at large, internal vehicles such as newsletters, payroll inserts, and educational sessions can be very effective. The people who comprise the sales and management staff will require more in-depth education as leaders of the effort.

There are fine lines to walk in cross-training for the continuum. For example, if you are operating in cost-based units with dedicated marketing representatives, they should be prepared for questions regarding other services and be able to direct the inquiries to another area for follow-up. However, they are dedicated to the unit and in general should not be considered to be continuum marketers.

While some hospitals and systems are choosing to begin sales cross-training and business development meetings, other corporate systems are mandating them. We met with hospital representatives and those who set the agendas for cross training/sales meetings and the business referral development committee. Some hospitals have chosen to hold one meeting while others break this into two sessions with different attendees. Some pointers for your consideration in designing your own systems approach to this are as follows:

- Invite the necessary participants only. Time is money!
- Have an agenda and a time allotment. Be efficient. This is an investment of time and money. Spend it wisely.
- Even the best of teams will have naysayers. The complaints will clear more quickly over time if management adheres to the first two tips and makes the time a worthwhile investment.
- Set the time strategically. Do not waste precious contact time. Avoid peak contact times for your locale. These usually include: 8 to 9:30 A.M., when offices are opening and physicians are making rounds and then heading to offices—a peak time for physicians and office staffs. 11 A.M. to 1 P.M., the hours surrounding lunch, are when offices may agree to education over a meal or agree to see reps just before and after lunch.

Sample Agenda: Monthly Cross Training/Sales Agenda

   I.   Opening
  II.   Sales Topics
         A. Skills workshop (this may be a new program, tours, inquiries, role plays, etc.)

III. Weekly Individual Goals
  A. Calls
  B. Targeted plans for the upcoming week
IV. Assignments and Adjourn
  A. What areas to prepare to present on next week, plans for special events, marketing plan preparation, etc.

This agenda works best for a relatively small number of participants (approximately seven to ten). Individual call reports and target profile reports may take longer with larger groups. Manage the time well. Do not allow this to monopolize all of the time allotted to reporting. Stress that this is for highlights only. Watch the team closely. If reps ramble in giving a report, they also may be rambling when conducting their one-to-one contacts and need assistance. In addition to this didactic approach to "sales training," you may also want to consider establishing rotation schedules for representatives through the other specialty areas or departments. Many facilities find this "walk a mile in my shoes" approach to be particularly effective (refer to Chapter 11).

Schedules to familiarize someone with a partial hospitalization program for geropsychiatric care might look like these two:

Admissions/Marketing Representative Briefing for Overview of Program and Materials to Read

- A.M.—Program participants arrive.—Observe the program in action throughout the day.
- Afternoon—Scheduled one-to-one calls with program representative.

Inpatient Rehabilitation

- A.M.—Shadow an orthopedic patient through morning therapy sessions.
- Noon on—Shadow a neurologic patient from lunch through the end of the day.

Any day spent shadowing a patient or provider will be helpful to demonstrate the types of patients and the actual flow of the program, whether through cardiac rehab, home health, or any other program. Select your "teacher" carefully; he or she must be willing to answer questions and educate your representatives.

Send representatives out with each other to mentor new or less experienced team members. However, as soon as the educational phase is completed, we suggest discontinuing this practice because it effectively cuts the effort in half. Program marketers may, of course, invite the program director along when it is indicated by the level of clinical expertise of the individual being contacted. Some groups even have a features-and-benefits sheet developed for each department. Each team member develops and presents the sheets. In addition each team member has a notebook with all of this information, so that he or she can review it before going out on a call.

Each member is given assignments to complete within the next month and will be asked to report back to the group. This usually includes one "sales" assignment and also individual call assignments to construct profile sheets on physicians. The profile sheets are submitted and maintained in a central file in administration so that anyone can refer to the sheets prior to leaving to conduct a contact meeting.

Business Development Meeting

I. Call to order

II. Old business—updates on managed care contracting, physician recruitment

III. New business

   A. One-to-one contacts

   B. Planned events

   C. Changes within the market (competitors, etc.)

IV. Assignments and adjourn

CONTACT PLANNING AND ROTATION SCHEDULES

Depending upon how the contacts are divided, the first step is to refer to the information from the management information system database and stratify targets. We recommend prioritizing the lists of targets into three areas:

Continuum Admitters: These more loyal physicians, or other referral sources, require relationship maintenance and might benefit from some "fine tuning" on identifying additional appropriate patients or nuances of the continuum (such as SNU for observation and monitoring or oversight of the home health care plan).

Program Admitters: This group may use only certain programs and not others. The object of the effort here is to determine if these referral sources could use additional continuum services to benefit their patients (for example, some patients that a physician refers to rehab who might be better served by home health).

Unknown Potentials: Because of their specialty or lower number of admissions, it is difficult to determine how the hospital's continuum services may be perceived by the referral source. The objective is to determine the potential and either remove the individual from the target list entirely or move them to another group eventually.

Rotation Schedules

While virtually anyone can conduct one-to-one calls, it takes careful planning to conduct an effective effort. We recommend that rotation schedules be established for planning purposes. This includes taking all of the information available regarding potential contacts and constructing a basic skeleton rotation schedule of who needs to be seen and how frequently. Unfortunately, in sales we sometimes see contacts who are friendly and nice to us but who never seem to refer. In fact, they might be moving their practice to another hospital!

As managers, we must constantly revise our plans and compare information regarding admissions to our goals. If someone is unhappy and stops referring, go find out why. Conversely, if someone begins to refer, say thank you and ascertain if the process is smooth. Whether the news is good or bad, the call has been a success.

We encourage you to develop a rotation schedule to fit your needs. If your facility or system has multiple representatives calling on the medical staff, they should share their rotation schedules at the meetings so that your referral sources are not bombarded by multiple representatives within a few days. Because there is success in moving referral sources up the ladder (or off the ladder), rotation schedules will change. Also the rotation schedule does not take into account the hallway meeting that may occur while a physician is making rounds at the hospital, thus allowing a rep to eliminate a call if follow-up does not warrant one. Be considerate of referral sources. They are busy people, too.

Evaluating and Monitoring the Effort

The one-to-one direct education contact effort should be continuously monitored, just as the hospital's promotional effort should be monitored. The following are our recommendations for the management of the direct effort.

Meet with the representative who is responsible for the effort on a weekly basis and review the past week's contacts (read their contact sheets), their outcomes, information gathered, and the written plans for the upcoming week's contacts. The important points to cover are:

- Who is being contacted and why? (Sometimes it is easier to call on those who we like, but they cannot always offer referrals.)
- What one-to-one contacts are planned?
- What special events or projects are in progress?
- How many referrals were received, and how many of these were admitted?
- What follow-up is necessary on your part? Is there any indication for follow-up that needs to be routed to another individual or department?

It is also highly recommended that you ride along once monthly with the individual on calls. This should be a spontaneous event to provide an accurate picture of what type of daily schedule the individual has. If the marketing professional has never done sales before yet manages the effort, this will develop not only knowledge but also empathy.

Invest time into thoroughly studying a book on sales management and sales techniques, or attend a seminar. You don't have to have all of the answers to gain the respect of those who are in the field, but you should have a basic understanding of what they do and the challenges they face.

In summary: To lead the team, the marketing manager must have in-depth knowledge of the targets and corresponding strategies. For maximum success, choose the right people to lead the effort, both internally and externally, and monitor the effort continuously.

Conclusion

"A heavy emphasis on the promotional aspects of marketing, with little or no appreciation for marketing's analytical and strategic bases, led many healthcare organizations to pursue strategies that wasted resources, and produced mediocre results or no results at all."[1]

Just as the delivery of healthcare itself has changed, so has the marketing and promotion of these services. Direct care providers have found themselves doing more with less and often must learn some tasks traditionally associated with other healthcare providers. Just as these specialists have diversified, so have marketers. From public relations to advertising, physician relations, business development, sales and managed care, we have also grown and changed.

Development of the continuum of care poses perhaps our greatest challenge yet. We now must be familiar with service components on a quasi-clinician level to question the system. At first glance, promotion of the components appears straightforward, but the internal systems of the organizations can affect the results of our marketing and call the results of our efforts into question. As professionals we must question not only our strategies and systems but also those of the organization in our search for success.

Our search for success led us to question hospital-based referral sources. We have surveyed those individuals performing discharge planning in various cities and continue to do so on an ongoing basis to collect information regarding the continuum of care. We would like to share some of the questions and the most frequent responses.

■ Do you believe that patients have any understanding of the continuum concept—"Quality Care provided in a more cost-effective setting?"

This question elicited an overwhelming "No." The responses indicate that patients only know they must leave the hospital sooner and do not understand the differences or regulations within the levels of care during a transition from acute care to home.

■ Are continuum services offered at the same location by providers and is this a factor in making referrals?

Responses to our question indicated that few providers offer the spectrum, but when they do it is definitely a factor in making referrals.

---

1. "American College of Health Care Executives Tutorial for the Governors Examination in Healthcare Management", The American College of Health Care Executives, 1997, Chicago, IL, page 50.

Several stipulated that the continuum offering will result in the provider being named as the first referral option. Provision of the continuum of care within a specialty program will even encourage individuals to cross geographic boundaries, because they perceive superior care.

■ Has there been or is there a significant level of advertising in your area regarding the continuum of care services to educate the public or does this occur through discharge planning?

To date, no responses have indicated continuum advertising. The inference is that organizations continue to position themselves as service component providers, not continuum providers. (You may have seen advertising by providers, but ask yourself: Is it programmatically continuum-focused or general advertising?)

Responses indicate that the discharge planning function is primarily responsible for this patient education with physicians and some specialty marketers becoming involved.

■ What is the role of the family in the continuum referral process?

Our responses indicate that the family makes the decision from the options available, unless the process is driven by managed care. (Increasingly, we are seeing the managed care component mentioned in response to this question.) Families are likely to select providers on the basis of reputation, advertising, word of mouth, location, convenience and insurance coverage.

■ "What are the roles of physicians and insurers in the referral process?"

Responses stipulate that insurers are involved if they have case management departments or contracts that direct referrals and specify network providers. Physicians influence the process by specifying the facility or level of care and by attending the patient at certain facilities where they are on staff or choose to make rounds.

These responses indicate that marketers have more challenges to face in continuum promotion. Just as continuum components work together to effectively treat the patient in the most efficient setting, we must internally process and externally promote efficiently. Whether this is the intake and tour process, discharge planning process, or territory and contact management, the focus is the same. By understanding our internal processes and intricacies of the products, we can market more effectively and successfully build revenues for the organization.

This book has put the tools into your hands. Remember, you can build anything if you have the right tools.

About the Author

Vicki Mason is a principal in Mason White & Associates in Dallas, Texas. The firm provides market analysis, marketing and communication services to the healthcare industry.

Ms. Mason is a frequent speaker whose engagements include the Healthcare Financial Management Association, the National Managed Care Congress and the Alliance for Health Care Strategy and Marketing. Her articles and comments have appeared in such publications as the *American Subacute Care Association Newsletter*, *Health Care Marketing Report* and in the book *Subacute Care* by Thompson Publishing.

Ms. Mason is a former clinician with 10 years of hospital experience. Her marketing career began in 1986 and has included positions in physician relations as director, regional director, and corporate marketing director, as well as vice president of corporate services, and chief marketing officer for hospitals and healthcare corporations. She holds a nursing facility administrator license and has completed courses for assisted living management certification. She received her master's degree in Health Services Administration from the College of St. Francis in Joliet, Illinois and an undergraduate degree from Murray State University in Murray, Kentucky.

INDEX